THE HEALing REVOLUTION DIET

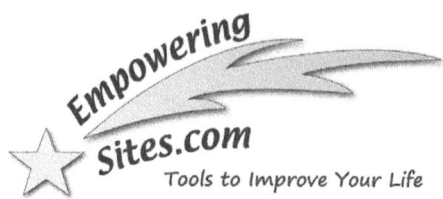

The HEALing Revolution Diet:
A Science-based Approach to Heal Your Gut, Reverse Chronic Illnesses,
Lose Weight, Clear Your Mind, and Increase Longevity

EmpoweringSites.com
Copyright © 2025 Randall S. Hansen, Ph.D.

All rights reserved. No part of this publication may be reproduced, distributed, or transmitted in any form or by any means, including photocopying, recording, or other electronic or mechanical methods, without the prior written permission of the publisher, except in the case of brief quotations embodied in critical reviews and certain other noncommercial uses permitted by copyright law.

To request permissions,
contact the publisher at ceo@empoweringsites.com

Ebook: 979-8-9872520-4-8
Paperback: 979-8-9872520-5-5

Library of Congress Control Number: 2024912727

Edited by Jenny Hansen, M.A.
Designed by Michelle Fairbanks

This book has been written for informational and educational purposes only. It is not intended to serve as medical advice, a substitute thereof, or a guarantee of outcome and should not be construed as such. It is always recommended to consult your healthcare provider for guidance on any aspect of medical treatment and care. Any use of the information in this book is based on the reader's judgment and is the reader's sole responsibility.

THE HEALING REVOLUTION DIET

A SCIENCE-BASED APPROACH to Heal Your Gut, Reverse Chronic Illnesses, Lose Weight, Clear Your Mind, and Increase Longevity

DR. RANDALL S. HANSEN, PH.D.
AUTHOR OF THE *WHOLEISTIC HEALING REVOLUTION TRILOGY*

DEDICATION

This book is dedicated to all those who are suffering because of our poor food system, incorrect nutrition information, and the cultural fixation on diet and appearance.

This book is for all of us who are diet survivors!

Please remember: *Food can truly be our medicine – but we need to be eating the RIGHT foods to make it true – otherwise, food becomes our poison.*

CONTENTS AT A GLANCE

Author's Note 1
Introduction 6
Health Assessment 12
Timeline of Our Food & Health Demise 14

PART ONE:
FOOD AS MEDICINE… NOT POISON

Chapter 1: The Healing Revolution Diet 22
Chapter 2: The Big Picture: It's Not You, It's the Food 41
Chapter 3: What "Foods" You Need to Eliminate 50
Chapter 4: What Foods You Should Be Eating 60
Chapter 5: How to Supplement Your Diet With Healthy Support 73
Chapter 6: Supporting Healthspan and Longevity –
  Sleep, Stress, Home, Community/Loneliness, Devices 80
Chapter 7: Wholeistic Healing…Why and How Health is More Than Just Food .. 94
Chapter 8: Health, Nutrition, and Diet Frequently Asked Questions (FAQ) 103
Chapter 9: Health, Nutrition, and Diet Do's and Don'ts 138

PART TWO:
HEALING REVOLUTION DIET TOOLS

Chapter 10: Healthy and Easy Recipes 144
Chapter 11: Top Tips from Expert Nutritionists/Dietitians 186

PART THREE:
HEALTH, NUTRITION, AND DIET SUCCESS STORIES

Chapter 12: David's Story 195
Chapter 13: Jake's Story 201
Chapter 14: Kali's Story 207
Chapter 15: Chris' Story 214
Chapter 16: Mandy's Story 220
Chapter 17: Emily's Story 226
Chapter 18: Susan's Story 232
Chapter 19: Shilpa's Story 238

PART FOUR:
HEALING REVOLUTION RESOURCES

Health, Nutrition, and Diet Resources 246
Health, Nutrition, and Diet Glossary 265
End Notes/Acknowledgements 275

EXPANDED CONTENTS

CHAPTER 1: THE HEALING REVOLUTION DIET

It's Not Just About Food and Diet 25
The Healing Revolution Diet 26
How Agriculture and Food Production Have Radically Changed in the Past Century 28
Nutrition and Food Myths Debunked 31
A Short History of Diets and Dieting... 35
Don't Overlook the Role of Obesogens 36
Cancers Specifically Associated With Excess Weight and Obesity 38
Moving Forward With the Healing Revolution Diet 39

CHAPTER 2: THE BIG PICTURE: IT'S NOT YOU, IT'S THE FOOD

What You Need to Know About the Gut Microbiome 42
What You Need to Know About Mitochondria 45
Our Food Choices Affect the Gut Microbiome and our Mitochondria 46
Your Role in the Big Picture of Health 47
A Final Word on Antibiotics and Other Medications 47

CHAPTER 3: WHAT "FOODS" YOU NEED TO ELIMINATE

The Ten Dangerous Foods/Ingredients to Eliminate From Your Diet 51
It's the Processing That's Literally Killing Us 54
Symptoms of a Sugar/Food Addiction 55
Breaking the Sugar/Food Addiction 55
Alternative Names for Sugar 58
A Final Word About Conventionally Raised Animals 59

CHAPTER 4: WHAT FOODS YOU SHOULD BE EATING

Why We Need to Reimagine Our Food Priorities 60
The Dangerous Nutrition Guidance from the U.S. Government 62
The Healing Revolution Food Pyramid 64
Breaking Down the Healing Revolution Food Pyramid 65
Tips for Getting Started on the Healing Revolution Diet 71
Final Thoughts on the Healing Revolution Diet 72

CHAPTER 5: HOW TO SUPPLEMENT YOUR DIET WITH HEALTHY SUPPORT

Major Categories of Dietary Supplements 75
Adaptogen Supplements 77
Dr. Randall's Personal List of Dietary Supplements 79
A Final Word About Supplements 79

CHAPTER 6: SUPPORTING HEALTHSPAN AND LONGEVITY – SLEEP, STRESS, HOME, COMMUNITY/LONELINESS, DEVICES

The Importance of Sleep to Health 81
The Importance of Safely Dealing With Stress 82
The Importance of Removing Household Toxins to Health 83
The Importance of Fortifying Healthy, Positive, and Loving Relationships 84
The Importance of Creating Strong Boundaries With Electronic Devices and Screens 85
The Importance of Practicing Forgiveness of Yourself and Others 86
The Importance of Daily Movement/Exercise 87
The Importance of Meaningful Work 88
The Importance of Establishing a Daily Gratitude Routine 89
The Importance of Practicing Self-Care 90
Wrapping It Up: The Importance of Healthspan and How to Accomplish It 91

CHAPTER 7: WHOLEISTIC HEALING... WHY AND HOW HEALTH IS MORE THAN JUST FOOD

How Do We Heal? 95
Trauma Assessment 101
A Final Word About Healing 102

CHAPTER 8: HEALTH, NUTRITION, AND DIET FREQUENTLY ASKED QUESTIONS (FAQ)

1. What's the best diet to follow – to lose weight? For longevity? 104
2. What's the best balance of carbs, fat, and protein in my diet? 105
3. Isn't fat bad for you, especially for your heart? 106
4. Sugars are carbs, which are needed, right? How bad is sugar – really? 107
5. What are the best/worst oils to use in cooking/baking? 108
6. Is meat bad for you? 109
7. Why should I pay more for organic produce? 110
8. What's the best source for healthy fresh foods? 111
9. What are ultra-processed foods, and why are they so bad? 112
10. How healthy is fast food? 113
11. What's wrong with conventionally grown fruits and vegetables? 114
12. Should I be following the U.S. government Food Pyramid or MyPlate? ... 115
13. Shouldn't I be counting calories if I am trying to lose or watch my weight? ... 116
14. What's the best way to ensure I am buying and eating healthy products? ... 116
15. Is it okay to eat snacks, especially if I eat smaller meals? 117
16. Can I skip breakfast? Isn't it called the most important meal of the day? ... 118
17. I don't have time to read the labels when I shop. Why should I bother? ... 119
18. I can't afford organic foods, what can I do? And why is healthy food so expensive? ... 120
19. I live in an area with limited access to quality foods, what can I do? 121
20. Why do some people say our food system is broken? 122
21. As long as I exercise regularly, I can eat whatever I feel like, right? 123
22. Should I go gluten-free or grain-free? 123
23. Should I go dairy-free? 124
24. What's the one thing I should eliminate from my diet today? 125
25. Should I be concerned about the lack of fiber in my diet? 126
26. Can my diet really help prevent diabetes, heart disease, cancer, and other chronic health conditions? 127
27. What role does hydration play in my health? 128
28. I don't have time to cook meals from scratch. What can I do? 129

29. I am afraid of fasting, is intermittent fasting a good option for me? 130
30. What are some simple ways I can improve my nutrition today? 131
31. What's up with all this talk about the gut microbiome? 132
32. Fermented foods seem really trendy, especially with longevity, are they healthy? 132
33. What is metabolic health and its relation to metabolic syndrome? 133
34. What are the best foods/diets for women in perimenopause and menopause? 135
35. Besides food, what other things can I be doing to improve my health? 136

CHAPTER 9: HEALTH, NUTRITION, AND DIET DO'S AND DON'TS

CHAPTER 10: HEALTHY, DELICIOUS, AND EASY HEALING REVOLUTION DIET RECIPES

Healthy, Hearty, and Easy Chili Recipe	146
Hearty and Healthy Crockpot Beef Recipe	147
Delightful and Spicy Thai Red Chicken Curry Recipe	148
Creamy, Nutritious Super Green Soup Recipe	149
Spicy and Smooth Coconut Carrot Soup Recipe	150
Healthy Beef Heart and Mushroom Stoup Recipe	151
Chunky Turkey Soup Provencal Recipe	152
Smooth Sweet Potato and Mushroom Soup Recipe	153
Kefir-Infused Chicken Stoup Recipe	154
Fast and Easy Spatchcock Roast Chicken Recipe	155
Delicious and Amazingly Simple Ran Burgers Recipe	156
Scrumptious and Simple Baked Chicken Breast Recipe	157
Mediterranean Tomato Almond Mushroom Chicken Strip Recipe	158
Super Easy and Delicious Trout Amandine Recipe	159
Magnificent Oven-Baked Macadamia-Encrusted Fish Recipe	160
Bountiful Bison Mouthwatering Meatball Recipe	161
Moist and Tasty Ground Turkey Mini Loaves Recipe	162
Deliciously Cheesy Oven-Baked Organic Eggs Recipe	163
Organic Crustless Keto Cheesy Quiche Recipe	164
Heavenly and Delicious Chicken Fricassee Recipe	165
Decadent and Delicious Waldorf Chicken Salad Recipe	166
Spicy Chicken Keto Taco Salad Recipe	167
Home-Style Smothered Meatball Casserole Recipe	168
Tasty and Simple Roasted Brussels Sprouts Recipe	169
Organic Buttermilk Ranch Salad Dressing Recipe	170
Tangy and Clean Thousand Island Salad Dressing Recipe	171

Delicious and Nutritious Crispy Kale Chip Recipe 172
Buttery Garlic-Infused Buttered Spinach Recipe 173
Nutritious and Mouthwatering Baked Sweet Potato Fries Recipe 174
Devilishly Delicious Keto Deviled Eggs Recipe 175
Tasty Treat Keto Almond Flour Waffle/Pancake Recipe 176
Delicious No-Sugar Classic Cheesecake Recipe 177
Sinfully Delicious Keto, No-Sugar Pecan Pie Muffin Recipe 178
Best Keto Delectable Chocolate Chip Cookie Recipe 179
Best Keto Holiday Sugarless "Sugar" Cookie Recipe 180
Nutritiously Yummy Sweet Potato Biscuit Cookie Recipe 181
Decadent and Simple Baked Pecan Snacks Recipe 182
Old Fashioned Baked Apples With Kefir Recipe 183
Hydrating and Refreshing Kefir Coconut Drink Recipe 184
Easy, Healthy, and Organic Vanilla Extract Recipe 185

AUTHOR'S NOTE

It's not you, it's the foods (and a few other key issues) that are making us fatter and sicker, whether you are aware of it or not. What we eat affects every function in our bodies – and brains – and our ability to lead a long and optimal life. Cancer, heart attacks, strokes, dementia – none of these things have to be in our future; it's not about genetics (well, a tiny bit), but mostly about how we treat our bodies and what we expose them to that determines our health – and healthspan.

Welcome reader! If you do not know my previous works related to healing and health or follow me on LinkedIn or through my websites, let me share some things that may help you decide if this is the book that is finally going to change every aspect of your life for the better.

I have been in the wellness space for more than two decades, starting the deep dive into the field when my own wellness started suffering. What I discovered shocked me, especially in terms of our food system and the quality of all the foods we produce for the Western diet. You may not believe me now, but keep reading and you will; the vast majority of foods available for purchase from most outlets are unhealthy… unhealthy for our bodies, brains, and gut.

While today it seems that many of the systems are working against our health and healing, I don't believe it was all a concerted effort to make us – and keep us – sick. There are certainly others who believe in a complete conspiracy by Big Chemical, Big Ag, Big Food, Big Pharma, Big Healthcare, Big Insurance, and Big Government… and they *could* be right.

As you'll learn when you read the book, the problems with our food began about 75 years ago, when President Dwight Eisenhower suffered a heart attack in office – the first president to fall ill to this condition. He survived the heart attack, but the incident set off a firestorm of activity to find out why heart disease was on the rise in the U.S. and what to do about it.

Unfortunately, the original research was flawed, and three-quarters of a century later, we are still paying the price with chronic mental and physical health issues. We are the sickest we have ever been as a population.

But this book encompasses so much more than just wellness – and it is certainly NOT another diet book (as that market is saturated). Plus, most of the diet books conflict with one another, adding to our confusion.

This book is about finding true healing – and optimal health – so you can live your happiest, longest, and healthiest life.

The cornerstone of this book is that we have lost our way with food, with eating. We are disconnected from nature, as well as the farmers and ranchers who grow our food. Food marketers mislead us all the time and the government not only has our food priorities backward, but the agencies that are supposed to protect our food system and promote the healthiest foods are corrupt and deeply influenced by the 12 or so companies that dominate all the foods and food brands in our supermarkets.

Food can be our medicine – or our poison – and I will clearly demonstrate to you which is which. If you are living with chronic health conditions, especially those that require a prescription, this book is for you.

If you are seeking a lifestyle to prevent chronic health conditions such as diabetes, high blood pressure, dementia and other neurodegenerative disorders, depression, anxiety, heart disease, and cancer, *this book is for you.*

If you are seeking to get off the diet hamster wheel of death and disease, this book is for you. And, yes, if you are looking to lose weight and keep it off, *this book is for you.*

My goal in writing this third book on healing is to help you discover how food can transform your life for the better – rather than the current situation, where the food you're eating is slowly (and painfully) killing you.

Life your BEST and HEALTHIEST life! Please join me – and many others – on the HEALING REVOLUTION!

A BIT ABOUT MY HEALTH JOURNEY

I grew up during a time when the food industry was much safer and better than it is today. I was also extremely lucky in that my mom cooked every meal, snack, and dessert from scratch. I only had cereal for breakfast if I stayed at a friend's house. I didn't even know that canned soup or bake mixes existed until I went to college.

But, from an early age, perhaps because of my mom's delicious desserts, I was a pudgy kid, stocky. I was never fat – because I was a very active kid, riding my bicycle everywhere – but I carried around that extra weight until my teenage growth spurt.

I had about a decade of being "slender" – at least in my eyes – but the stresses of adult life, career, and marriage and a family, led me to eating a lot of fast foods, convenience foods, and other junk foods. The marriage was not a good one, so food also became a comfort for me. I gained weight.

I spent about another decade trying every diet known… including some I made up. I almost always lost weight initially, as many do, but eventually gained it back, sometimes gained back more. Sometimes the diet stopped working, other times I had to cheat because I felt so deprived.

During that time, I was often sick – easily catching colds and the flu. Why? Because my immune system was compromised by the crappy, conventional foods I was eating. *I was metabolically unhealthy.*

But in my late 30s, I discovered something that changed my life, and that is partly why I am writing this book today. I learned that sugar is a toxin and seriously hurts the body, while also learning that sugar is a massive driver in weight gain (and many other serious health issues). I quit the sugary drinks and almost immediately lost 20 pounds. I cut out more sugar and lost more weight.

I then eliminated all white foods – flour and rice mainly – and fried foods. I lost more weight… *and kept it off.*

It wasn't all about food, though that was the main driver. I started walking and riding a bicycle again.

I also started reading labels – only to discover that sugar is hiding in most processed foods in the supermarket. I then started making my own salad dressing, my own tomato sauce. I found the rare companies that produced both organic and sugar-free products.

I also learned about the horrible way we industrially farm and ranch. With conventional farming, we are destroying the soil with the tilling and chemicals we use (in massive amounts) on the crops to increase yield, leaving us eating pesticide-laden foods. With conventional ranching, we are producing sick animals that must be given antibiotics; look at how chickens are raised or find pictures of cattle feedlots. It is absolutely sickening from an animal rights perspective – but also from a food and health perspective.

Finally, I learned about the lies behind fats. Many demonized animal fats as bad for heart health, and even though this was completely disproved (more than a decade ago), we still have people making this claim. Because of the push for "healthier" oils and because manufacturers had long been industrially processing seeds for oil, we are now awash in these dangerous oils. You'll learn that the vast majority of Americans get the highest amount of calories from soybean oil (which is often sold as "vegetable" oil).

Today, it is much easier to find small brands producing foods free of sugar, seed oils, and other dangerous chemicals and additives. There are also wonderful small farmers and ranchers producing high-quality and safe foods, regenerating the soil and treating their animals with love and respect. I will be highlighting some of these brands in this book.

All those years of dieting and gaining and losing weight also gave me a body image complex. Happily, with healing and an amazing partner, I am mostly over those issues. I also believe that most bodies have a happy equilibrium – a weight range that fits – so the goal is to find that and live with it. Not all of us are meant to be skinny, but none of us are meant to be obese or vastly overweight.

And I have to tell you: it's the broken food system that is making most people sick, overweight, suffering.

Companies use the cheapest ingredients as the base for their products – which means not only are the foods of questionable quality, but also filled with genetically-modified products, sugar, toxic oils, antibiotics, growth hormones, pesticides and herbicides, and other dangerous chemicals and additives.

I am living proof that you can change. I am living proof that you can fight the broken food system and win. I am living proof that you can transform your life, transform your health, with a change in what you eat and how you source your food. I am living proof that you can improve your health by simply changing your diet and making a few other lifestyle adjustments.

I want you to have my decades of personal experience combined with my years as a trained researcher and educator to help you succeed in your health journey. I love finding and exposing the TRUTH, and sharing the latest research with you.

We don't have to be sick, tired, depressed, and struggling with chronic health problems.

I also believe that each of us HAS to find the food/diet that works best for our bodies. There is NO ONE diet for everyone. Yes, for some keto might be best; for some, perhaps carnivore; for others, vegetarian or vegan; and for others, perhaps the Mediterranean Diet.

One thing to keep in mind as you read the book: Our guts are either our first or second brain, depending on the expert. Thus, please understand that every item we eat has a direct impact on our bodies, our immune systems, and our mental health.

One final word about longevity. My goal with this book is not longevity, though I think it is a side benefit. Longevity is wonderful, but who wants to live a long life dealing with chronic health conditions and pain? I think longevity is not as important as health and living a long and healthy life free of chronic health issues, which is why some of us are now discussing "healthspan," rather than just longevity.

Finally, remember that while healing your health and gut is extremely important, it is also important to heal from past trauma – which is the focus of my first two books – and I strongly encourage you to embark on a complete health and healing journey for the perfect equation to living your optimal and most joyful life.

Let's start with one small step today!!

Know that I am wishing you great success and abundant health, healing, and happiness. We have hope!

–DR. RANDALL
"HEALINGSEED.WORLD" HANSEN*

*Curious? Go to HealingSeed.World

INTRODUCTION

"All disease begins in the gut." Hippocrates, the father of modern medicine, stated this more than 2,000 years ago, and yet we're only listening to this advice now.

How's your health? I hate to break it to you, but you may be sicker than you think. According to the latest research, about 90 percent of Americans have metabolic health issues, which can lead to metabolic syndrome and a host of serious chronic health illnesses, such as heart disease, diabetes, cancer, neurodegenerative disorders, and stroke.

Note: You can look healthy on the outside, but unfortunately NOT be healthy on the inside.

I encourage you to take the health assessment following this introduction and make an honest assessment of your mental and physical health.

I was part of that 90 percent with metabolic health issues for about half my life; I had blood sugar, cholesterol, and triglyceride issues. It affected my mental health as well. I looked healthy on the outside, but was sick on the inside.

We've been led to believe that many of our biggest chronic illnesses – the top killers today – are either random acts of disease or perhaps hereditary. But we are discovering that the vast majority of chronic conditions – diabetes, dementia, heart disease, stroke, and many cancers – are PREVENTABLE (and if caught early enough, reversible).

Food can either be our medicine… or our poison. And for the last four to five decades, as food and eating patterns have evolved, the conventional foods found in the grocery aisles are slowly poisoning us, leading to the massive chronic health problems we face today.

Our conventional food system, including our understanding of nutrition and dieting, is defective. We have become too easily distracted by the dieting wars, the wide availability of prepared and fast foods (of questionable quality), and the attention focused on weight-loss drugs.

Sadly, even the basic ingredients of our foods have been adversely affected. Our poor (industrial) farming practices have stripped the soil of nutrients, resulting in fewer nutrients in our fruits and vegetables. Because of a strict focus on productivity, we have also seen a dramatic increase in toxic chemicals (pesticides, herbicides, and fertilizers) sprayed onto our foods and absorbed into our bodies.

Furthermore, most of us are also on one or more prescription medications – and many of these drugs slow or block our ability to absorb what little nutrients are still in our foods.

The information in this book is going to blow open all the dirty food and diet lies in an effort to set you free to focus on what matters most: your health and the health of your loved ones. My goal is to educate and empower you!

This book is based on all the latest research from the best academics and doctors in the field – research that has not been influenced by the food industry's deep pockets, which you'll learn about in future chapters.

Many of us are literally eating ourselves to death. It's so bad, we even have an acronym for it: SAD (Standard American Diet), which consists of ultra-processed foods, with added sugars and salts, artificial flavors and colorings, refined/bleached grains, as well as toxic fats and oils. About 50 percent of the calories in SAD come from simple carbohydrates! Missing from SAD are fresh fruits, vegetables, healthy proteins, healthy fats, and whole grains.

Unfortunately, it is no longer just the Standard American Diet. The U.S. marketers have spread their cheap foods across the globe, resulting in some people referring to it now as the Standard Global Diet, making the entire world become sicker.

There are multiple indicators of the problems/implications with our food system and the "foods" we consume:

- Obesity (now at the highest levels ever)
- Type 2 diabetes (at epidemic levels)
- Cardiovascular/heart disease

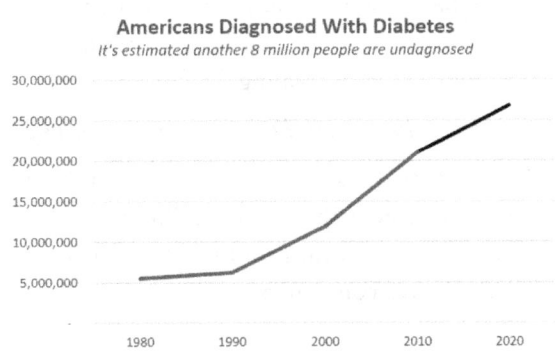

- Brain fog/memory issues/dementia
- Hypertension
- Strokes
- Cancers
- Liver diseases
- Kidney/gallbladder disorders
- Osteoarthritis
- Gastroesophageal reflux disease (GERD)

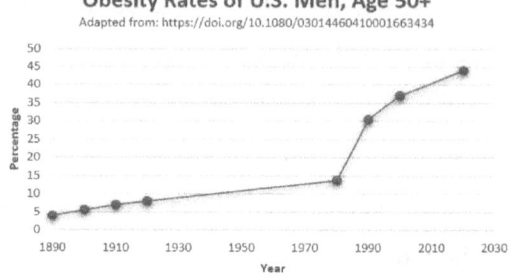

How concerned should we be? The World Obesity Federation's 2023 atlas predicts that 51 percent of the world, or more than 4 billion people, will be obese or overweight within the next 12 years – with the rates of obesity rising quickly among children and in lower income countries.

Within the U.S., the obesity rate has exploded since the 1980s, as shown on this chart. What happened in the 1970s that led to the rise in obesity, diabetes, and other chronic illnesses?

- High fructose corn syrup (HFCS), with a higher amount of the toxic element fructose, replaces sugar in many foods and beverages;
- Glyphosate (brand name Roundup), a dangerous chemical herbicide with links to cancer, sold commercially everywhere;
- Margarine, made with dangerous artificial trans fats at the time, reaches the height of sales, before scientists start questioning its safety;
- *Dietary Goals for the U.S.* was published by Congress, which stresses that sugar and carbohydrates are healthy and fat is bad – the complete opposite of the truth as we know it.

Sorry to be the one who has to tell you this, but in order to heal and live your best and healthiest life, you will have to relearn and rethink almost everything you know about trauma, healing, health, food, diet, exercise, and more.

The Healing Revolution Diet is a transformative lifestyle.

We have been (mostly) unintentionally misled into thinking we have the best – the best of everything – including the best food system, the best healthcare system, the best farming and ranching operations, the best restaurants, the best pharmaceutical companies.

Sadly, the United States is far from the best in most categories.

This book is about changing your mind, changing your actions, changing your life – for the better.

One of my favorite comments about my books is that I do not take a dogmatic approach; instead, I present the facts – and the TRUTH – and let you decide, and the same holds true for this book.

I do have a few hard and fast rules for you, but it is NOT about dieting or weight loss or having to choose a side in the crazy "diet wars" of vegan versus carnivore versus keto versus…

My goal is for you to find your way – the way that works for your body and your lifestyle. No dietary advice fits all people, and if you get anything from this book, please get this: Your goal should be finding a food/nutrition plan that works for YOU – not just for today, but for the rest of your life, being open to modifying the mix based on your circumstances.

Too many people jump on one of the many big or fad diets and find some initial success, but then often find themselves cheating because the diet is too restrictive or simply because the diet stops working for them… often leading to weight gain, and what experts call yo-yo dieting.

With this book and plan, there will be no more bouncing from one weight to another, moving from one set of clothing to the next, based on your weight loss/gain. Also, no more weighing yourself daily – nor weighing your foods. No more counting calories or points.

What I hope to leave you with is a lifestyle plan, not a diet plan. A nutrition plan, not a calorie-restrictive plan. A healthspan and longevity plan, not a life with chronic illness plan.

This plan will help you improve your health, improve your life. This plan will help you wean off pharmaceuticals you may already be taking because of chronic illnesses. This plan will improve your mental and physical health. This plan is truly PREVENTATIVE, for a better, healthier, and longer life.

This plan will take hard work and a commitment to health and healing. It will take massive changes to your understanding of food and health. It will be challenging at times and you will be *fighting* a food system that is indifferent to human *and* animal health, as long as consumers are buying their products and the profits keep rolling in.

And it's NEVER too late to start this plan. While it's ideal to start as soon as possible – for you and your loved ones (and especially young children) – the goal is to START. Start implementing just one thing from the following pages today, and build on that in the coming weeks and months.

All that said, once you implement this plan, start actively living this plan, you will emerge with the best health of your life, healing your gut, and healing your brain.

Besides all the most current research and truthful information about food, health, nutrition, and diet, this book also includes stories from people who have transformed their lives through healthier eating. My hope is you'll be inspired and empowered by one or more of the stories to start and continue on your health and healing journey.

The later section of the book includes some simple recipes to assist you and inspire you. Cooking and baking from scratch can be fun, exciting, and something everyone can participate in. My recipes are not gourmet and will never win any epicurean awards, but they are designed to have the highest nutrition while making preparation fairly easy and cooking times short – because these recipes are designed for busy people who don't have hours every day to spend on shopping, prepping, and cooking meals.

Finally, to assist you in your healing, and to break up some of the text, I am including a variety of additional information, tips, advice, and quotes using the following techniques:

AUTHOR INSIGHTS: Interesting and informative food, diet, nutrition, and healing tidbits the author wants to highlight.

INSPIRING QUOTES: Short, motivating, and/or thought-provoking passages related to food, diet, nutrition, and healing from a range of people and experts.

FOOD FACTS: Nugget-sized bits of fascinating, critical data, truths, or history about food, diet, nutrition.

HEALING HINTS: Concise blurbs of expert advice to assist/help you further understand healing, nutrition, and food.

One final note: I have no agenda here besides seeing you heal. I have no paid program or coaching. I am simply in service of helping the world heal – in helping YOU heal.

Going to the supermarket should not feel like work... or worse, like a maze in which you struggle trying to find the healthiest foods for you and your loved ones. Do be forewarned, the typical grocery store is filled with marketing traps to confuse and frustrate you.

This book provides you with all the tools to succeed in finding the best foods for your health and healing!

EDITORIAL NOTE: *Some of the work in this book requires changing lifestyles, deep breathing, new foods, and other changes that might put a strain on your body. It is highly recommended that you receive support from a doctor (ideally a naturopath) before jumping into a new healing regimen. None of this work is dangerous for the healthy individual, but it's important to always be safe... especially since our goal is healing and living a joyous and authentic life. And if your current doctor does not support your healing protocol, PLEASE consider finding a new doctor.*

The Supermarket Maze for Finding the Best Foods

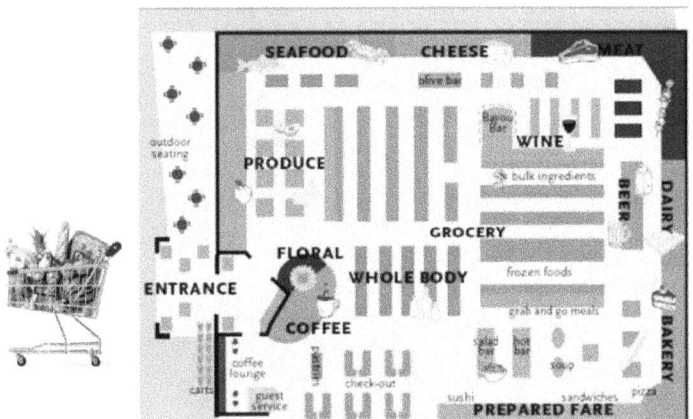

The KEY is buying only real foods, not ultra-processed.

HEALING REVOLUTION DIET HEALTH ASSESSMENT

This assessment is at the front of the book because the only way this book or any advice will help you is when you take an honest reflection on how you really feel. Our brains are quite good at ignoring signs and signals from the body that something is not right.

What you're currently eating, combined with other lifestyle factors, impacts your health more than you may realize. Health is not just about having an "ideal" weight, as many components of health lie just below the surface (literally) until a major crisis erupts.

How healthy are you? *Take this quick assessment.*

ANSWER YES OR NO TO THE FOLLOWING STATEMENTS:

I am dealing with...

1. Feeling over-committed and over-stressed — YES / NO
2. Ongoing weight gain; difficulty losing weight — YES / NO
3. Fluid retention; feeling puffy — YES / NO
4. Sessions of brain fog; trouble concentrating — YES / NO
5. Complacency; less empathy and compassion — YES / NO
6. Stomachaches; abdominal bloating — YES / NO
7. Feelings of being overwhelmed; anxious — YES / NO
8. Difficulty with sleep; not able to get good rest — YES / NO
9. A sense of burnout; overly aggressive at times — YES / NO
10. Having sugar, carb, or alcohol cravings — YES / NO
11. One or more addictions (food, porn, gambling, etc.) — YES / NO

12. Times of fatigue; feeling tired most of the time	YES	NO
13. Minimal bowel movements; less than once a day	YES	NO
14. Too many bowel movements; diarrhea	YES	NO
15. Being sick more often than others; catch every cold/flu	YES	NO
16. Mood swings that have grown more severe	YES	NO
17. Inflamed gums, bleeding gums, cavities, root canals	YES	NO
18. Cracked lips, also known as "cheilitis."	YES	NO
19. Hair changes; hair dry like straw	YES	NO
20. New allergies	YES	NO

SCORING: Give yourself 1 point for every "yes" response. If you score more than 3, your health is under attack and you need to take action to start healing. You need the advice in this book… keep reading!

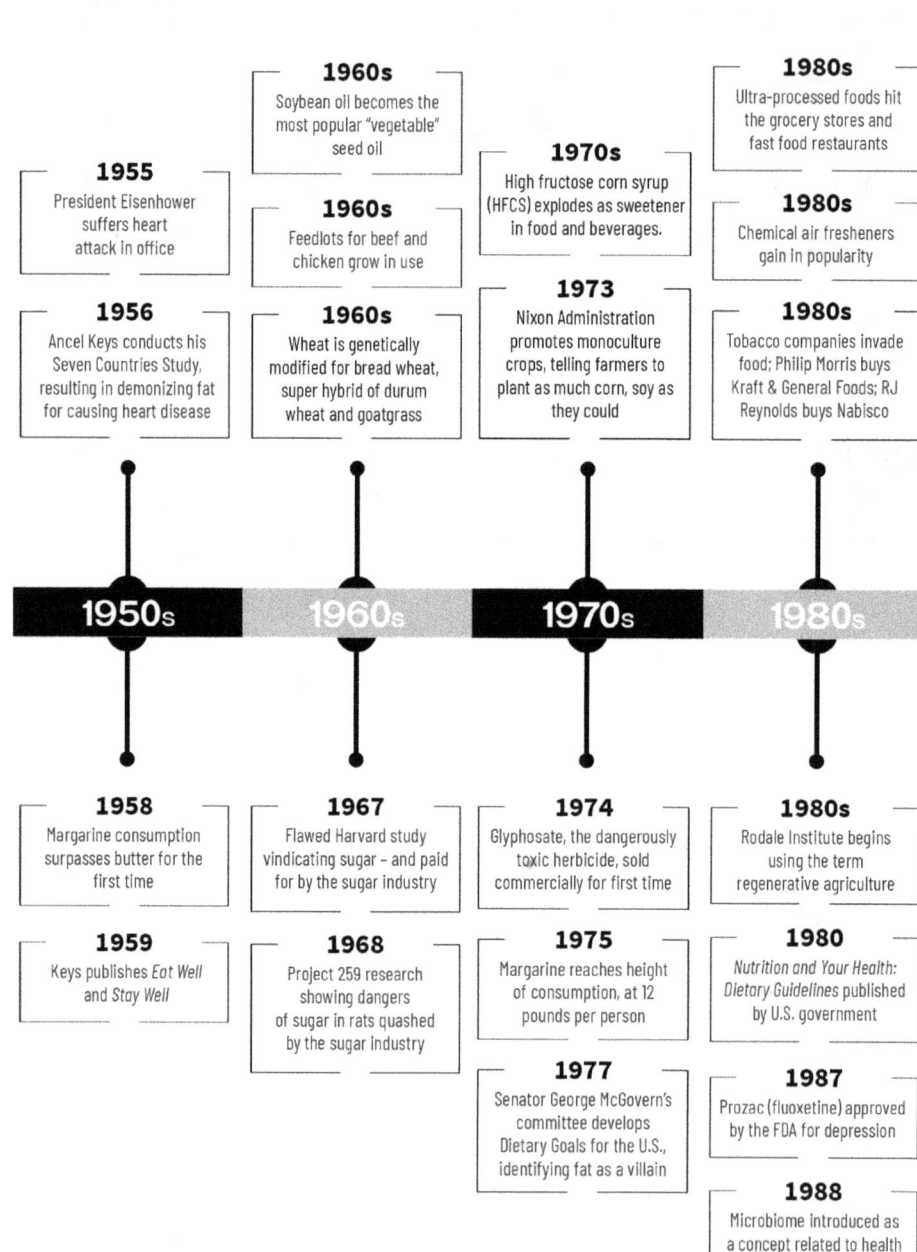

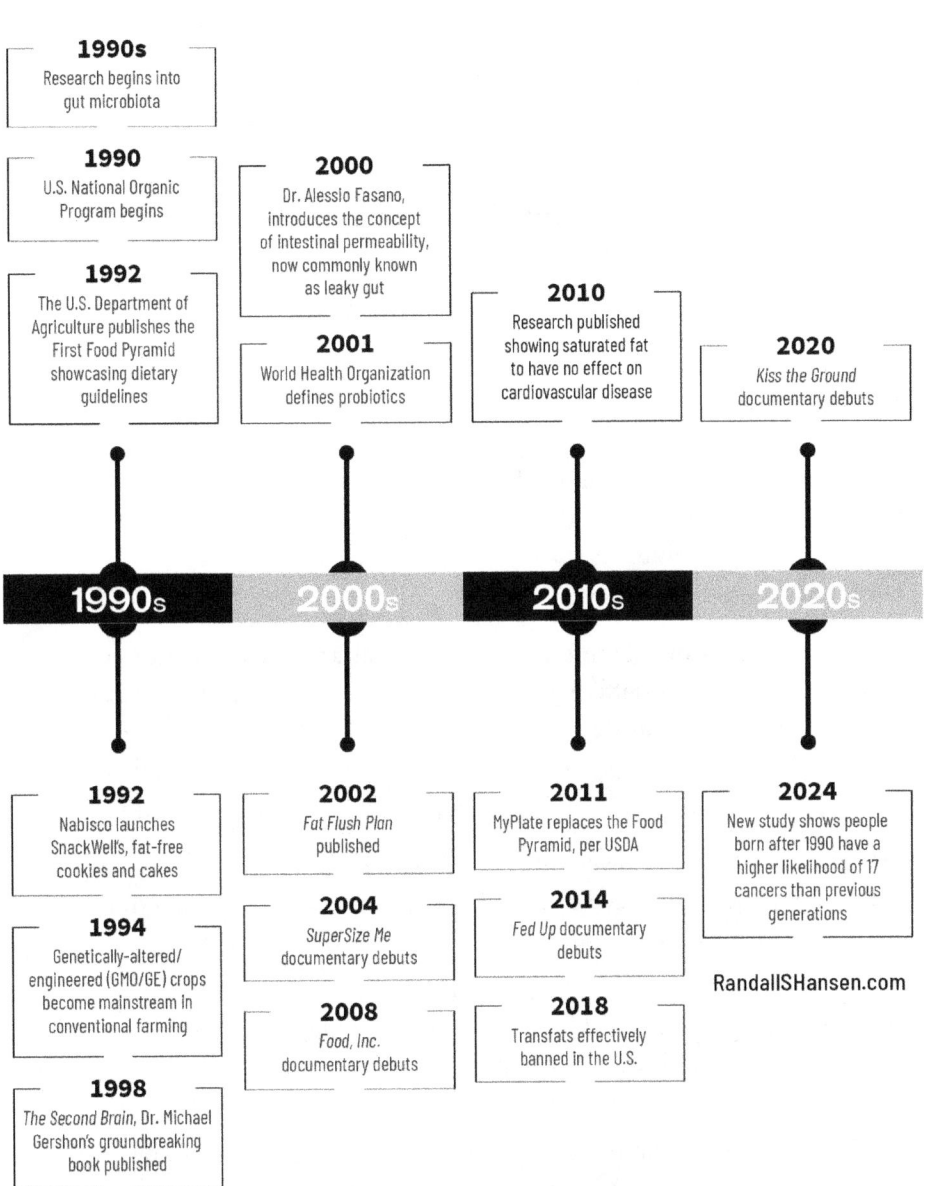

What has happened in the past 75 years to so radically change the health of most of the Western world, and now even into many developing countries?

IT'S THE FOOD. It's everything about the food, from the types of foods we are now growing and producing to the types of convenience foods we are now eating for many meals. It's the vast increase in sugar in all food products, the prevalence of cheap seed oils in place of healthy fats, and the vast amount of added chemicals (from pesticides in the growing to preservatives and emulsifiers in the final product) in our food system.

Please review this timeline of events that have had a direct influence on our food and nutrition. Included are key events from:

- Chemical Industry
- Healthcare Industry
- Pharmaceutical Industry
- Food Industry
- Farming Practices
- Governmental Policies and Subsidies
- Health Agencies
- Documentary Films
- Groundbreaking Authors

We are suffering from the most serious physical and mental health crisis ever seen. Many people are suffering from insulin resistance, diabetes, heart disease, dementia, and cancer, as well as struggling with weight and obesity. A growing number of people are struggling with anxiety, depression, OCD, addiction.

Here are some of the major milestones that have led to declining healthspan.

1955: President Eisenhower suffers a heart attack while in office, triggering near-hysteria over this new disease affecting more and more Americans. This event started a "contest" for researchers to uncover what was causing this deadly disease.

1956: Ancel Keys conducts his Seven Countries Study, resulting in demonizing fat for causing heart disease; years later, researchers reviewing his work find that sugar actually has a much higher correlation to heart disease than fat.

1958: Margarine consumption surpasses butter for the first time, showcasing the progress of seed oils over natural, healthy fats, and the beginning of decades of fearing beneficial fats while replacing them with cheap and dangerous products made from seed oils.

1959: Ancel Keys publishes *Eat Well and Stay Well,* which stressed the "dangers" of fat in affecting people's hearts, arteries, and blood cholesterol levels. He adamantly defended his research to the point of bullying any researcher who questioned his misguided findings.

1960s: Wheat is genetically modified for bread wheat, a super hybrid of durum wheat and goatgrass, which leads to much greater yields and profits, but greatly impacts the quality. Experts say this change is part of the problem with some gluten sensitivities.

1960s: Feedlots for beef and chicken grow in use, resulting in the industrialization of meat production. With feedlots come pollution and environmental issues, animal welfare concerns, and the beginning of a massive increase in the use of cheap grain feed, as well as routine administering of antibiotics and growth hormones.

1960s: Soybean oil becomes the most popular "vegetable" seed oil, used in many ultra-processed packaged and fast foods because of its extremely low cost to food manufacturers thanks to U.S. government subsidies. Soybean oil is also often labeled as "vegetable" oil.

1967: Flawed Harvard study vindicating sugar as safe – and paid for by the sugar industry. The impact of this study reinforced the finding from Keys, until decades later when the sugar funding was discovered. Furthermore, the fallout from this study reinforced the importance of always examining what entities provided the funding for food research studies.

1968: Project 259, research showing serious dangers of sugar in rats, is quashed by the sugar industry – and buried for decades until the truth was eventually discovered.

1973: The Nixon Administration promotes monoculture crops, telling farmers to plant as much corn, soy as possible, further promoting the wrong crops and the worst type of farming.

1974: Glyphosate, the toxic herbicide, sold commercially for first time, fostering the beginning of a massive love affair with conventional farmers, who drench crops in it at least twice during the growing cycle.

1970s: High fructose corn syrup (HFCS) explodes as a sweetener in food and beverages because of its cheap cost compared to refined sugar, because corn is highly subsidized by the U.S. government.

1975: Margarine reaches height of consumption, at 12 pounds per person.

1977: Senator George McGovern's committee develops *Dietary Goals for the U.S.*, identifying fat as a villain, beginning the government's deeper involvement in recommending nutrition and food guidelines.

1980: *Nutrition and Your Health: Dietary Guidelines* released by the U.S. Department of Agriculture (USDA) and Health and Human Services (HHS), stressing nutritional advice.

1980s: Ultra-processed foods hit grocery stores and fast food restaurants, forever changing the landscape of food production. Food scientists were hired to chemically alter food ingredients to make foods hyperpalatable – with pleasure points to hijack the brain and make the foods addictive.

1980s: Chemical air fresheners gain in popularity, adding to the ongoing onslaught of chemicals in the home, including toxic cleaners, laundry detergents, dryer sheets, and more.

1980s: Rodale Institute begins using the term "regenerative agriculture," a turning point for understanding how farming practices can enhance the soil rather than destroying it.

1980s: Tobacco companies invade food; Philip Morris buys Kraft & General Foods; RJ Reynolds buys Nabisco. Taking the marketing power from their success with cigarettes, these companies pushed for the development of hyperpalatable, addictive foods.

1987: Prozac (fluoxetine) approved by the FDA for depression, opening the door for the huge influx of antidepressants to hit the market. Unfortunately, these medications barely performed better than placebos and were only tested for short-term use; furthermore, they were developed with a now outdated theory that depression was due to a serotonin imbalance.

1988: "Microbiome" introduced as a concept related to health, which slowly opens the door to reexamining the gut as a key component of health.

1990: U.S. National Organic Program begins to help consumers navigate a growing problem of too many chemical residues on conventionally grown fruits and vegetables, drawing key distinctions and showing the benefits of buying organic.

1990s: Research begins into gut microbiota. Building on the concept of the gut microbiome, researchers dive deeper into all aspects of the gut and intestinal system.

1992: The U.S. Department of Agriculture publishes the First Food Pyramid showcasing dietary guidelines, further stepping into its role in educating consumers about the best daily food consumption. Unfortunately, these guidelines were completely wrong, misguided.

1992: Nabisco launches SnackWell's, fat-free cookies and cakes, which propels no-fat products as a top food category, with many other food marketers adding low-fat and no-fat products, which often have added sugar and numerous chemicals to make up for the fat.

1994: Genetically-altered/engineered (GMO/GE) crops become mainstream in conventional farming, mainly because they increased yield – and thus profits. Organic foods cannot contain any GMO ingredients.

1998: *The Second Brain*, Dr. Michael Gershon's groundbreaking book published, which focuses on the then-discovery of nerve cells in the gut acting as a "second brain," and coordinating with the brain in our head.

2000: Dr. Alessio Fasano, introduces the concept of intestinal permeability, now commonly known as *leaky gut*, with underwhelming response and questions; of course, we now know that leaky gut is a major driver in toxins entering the bloodstream.

2001: The World Health Organization defines probiotics as "live microorganisms which when administered in adequate amounts confer a health benefit on the host." Live probiotic cultures are part of fermented foods and probiotic-fortified foods, and are also available as supplements.

2002: *Fat Flush Plan*, by Dr. Ann Louise Gittleman, is published; a book that changed the course of the author's life. The plan focuses on increasing metabolism, flushing out bloat, speeding up fat loss, and decreasing inflammation, but the biggest takeaway was her demonization of processed sugar.

2004: *SuperSize Me* documentary debuts in which Morgan Spurlock, an American independent filmmaker, filmed his consumption of McDonald's food for 30 days. The results on his health in just that short period were shocking, though it has since been reported he was also heavily drinking during the filming.

2008: *Food, Inc.* documentary debuts, and for the first time, viewers get a firsthand account of the dangers of the industrial production methods used in the American food industry, with the film exploring how corporations place profits before consumer health, worker safety, and the environment.

2010: Research published showing saturated fat to have little to no effect on cardiovascular disease, ending decades of misinformation and incorrect nutritional guidance. If not fat? Sugar.

2011: MyPlate replaces the Food Pyramid, with the USDA attempting to appeal to consumers with a different image, but the same bad advice of eating lots of carbs and several glasses of dairy.

2014: *Fed Up* documentary debuts, which examines the obesity epidemic, including the associated problems of diabetes and heart disease. The filmmaker makes the case that ultra-processed foods, and specifically the massive amounts of added sugar, are a critical underlying cause of the health crisis.

2018: Transfats effectively banned in the U.S. Transfats are artificial, hydrogenated vegetable oils that have serious health consequences, including increased likelihood of heart disease. Transfats were an inexpensive substitute for butter and lard, and used in the production of cookies, crackers, bread, frozen foods and more; many restaurants used transfats for frying.

2020: *Kiss the Ground* documentary debuts, which makes the premise of the power of regenerative agriculture to help heal the world's soils, completely and rapidly stabilize the Earth's climate, restore lost ecosystems, and create abundant food supplies. It highlights the important role healthier soil plays.

2024: New study shows that people born after 1990 have a higher likelihood of 17 cancers than previous generations. These cancers are linked to poor diet (including the high amounts of sugars and seed oils along with the almost elimination of fiber), and include pancreatic, kidney and small intestine cancers.

FINAL THOUGHTS ON THE FOOD & HEALTH DEMISE TIMELINE

It's fairly clear from the timeline that our health crisis has been decades in the making, some of it perhaps by accident, but others driven purely by money – the focus on the cheapest ingredients, expanding yield in crops and animals at all costs, and the drive for profits over health consequences.

For people interested in improving health, in finding healing, there are decades of momentum to overcome – but it's possible. People are winning every day. They are winning by learning the truth about all these industries and companies working against us and by listening to their bodies and brains and guts – and eating only the best real foods that foster their health.

You can do it too! Don't be a victim any longer; you can be a survivor! You can have better health and a longer healthspan. Information and knowledge are the key.

Please keep reading…

PART ONE: FOOD AS MEDICINE... NOT POISON

THE HEALING REVOLUTION DIET

An Approach to Eating and Living Based on 10 Principles

1. Stop dieting, following diet fads
2. Eliminate refined sugar consumption
3. Focus on healthy fats and proteins
4. Greatly reduce ultra-processed foods, fast foods, and takeout
5. Cook more from scratch
6. Add more fiber, especially from vegetables and seeds and nuts
7. Eat regeneratively grown foods from local farms and ranches
8. Buy organic over conventionally grown foods
9. Grow your own food
10. Improve all aspects of your dieta/lifestyle

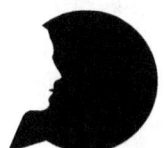

AUTHOR INSIGHT

Food can truly be our medicine – but we need to be eating the RIGHT foods to make it true – otherwise, food becomes our poison, damaging our guts, brain, heart, and immune system – and leading to a host of chronic illnesses.

CHAPTER ONE
The Healing Revolution Diet

This is **NOT** a diet book.

Perhaps it should be labeled the "anti-diet book."

The Healing Revolution Diet is a healing and transformative lifestyle, focused on an accurate and healthy understanding of health, healing, food, and nutrition. It is based on the premise that healthy foods can and should be the foundation for life, for living, and for longevity.

The number of mistakes, lies, and misinformation in the agriculture, food, pharmaceutical, healthcare, and nutrition industries over the past 70 years will stun you; it sure stunned me. How have we gotten food and health so wrong? Why are we the unhealthiest – mentally and physically – than we have ever been?

The answers to these questions will be unraveled in the pages of this book, but the questionable and unethical actions over the past 70 years would make a great horror movie, with plenty of villains and few heroes.

Once we understand the truths, we can move to having good health and living our optimal lives – and that is the premise and focus of the Healing Revolution Diet.

Because of the unhealthy foods and misguided food recommendations, many people have turned to diets and dieting, making it a multi-million dollar industry. We have been misled by the hundreds of diet plans and diet books. Almost all of the traditional diets are restrictive, which means people who try them are *set up to fail*… which leads to multiple consequences, including weight gain (typically after a short period of losing weight), shame, anger, frustration, and hopelessness.

Many of these diets fail. Why? Let's use the letters from the word DIET:

- **D**aunting
- **I**neffective
- **E**xasperating
- **T**iresome

And as one friend of mine likes to point out DIET is one letter away from DIE!

Very few diets are designed to be maintained over a lifetime; many are designed as short-term solutions, which is interesting because the root of diet in Latin is diaeta, meaning "prescribed way of life."

The Healing Revolution Diet is built to be a way of life, a way of living. It follows similar beliefs as the dieta used in traditional Ayahuasca healing ceremonies in which "dieta" refers to a set of life guidelines – which include food/diet, but go far beyond it to include all aspects of life and living.

Every aspect of the Healing Revolution Diet is based on the most current scientific and medical research and understanding, designed for lifetime use by anyone interested in health and healing, proven to help reverse chronic illnesses, and intended to help people live a longer healthspan (which is better than simply longevity).

FOOD FACT:
Humans are naturally adapted to an omnivorous diet because we have canine teeth meant for tearing into meat, as well as enzymes in our gut to digest animal protein and fats, states Barbara Kingsolver in *Animal, Vegetable, Miracle*.

You may be shocked at what you discover in these pages, including:

- Food companies producing and marketing products with unsafe (and often untested) additives and preservatives, favoring profits over people. These same handful of companies (about 12 in all) own the majority of *all* food brands sold (including organic brands), which gives them even more power to control the food system.

- Supermarkets and other grocery outlets and almost all fast food restaurants and takeout places selling dangerous "foods" in which most of the items sold are considered ultra-processed, removing beneficial ingredients while adding sugar and other addictive ingredients.

- Sugar companies lying to the public since the 1960s when their own research showed the dangerous side effects from consuming sugar, especially fructose.

- Agriculture companies raising (with financial subsidies from the U.S. government) huge amounts of chemically-produced monoculture crops that go directly into most of our foods, animal feed, and gasoline in the form of corn and soybeans, which accounts for 70 percent of all the planted farmland in the U.S.

- Conventional fruit and vegetable farms, also dominated by a few large companies, focusing entirely on efficiency and yield over healthy and safe crops... using a selection of chemicals to manage crop production, including fertilizers, pesticides, and herbicides. Most also use genetically-modified seeds designed not for taste but for maximizing yield.

- Government and health agencies promoting incorrect and harmful information based on old, outdated, and incorrect research and/or influenced by the huge amount of money spent by the major corporations in the form of political campaign contributions or sponsorships.

- Doctors and other healthcare professionals (who receive almost no nutritional education or training) providing inaccurate and wrong information, if anything at all.

- Healthcare providers who are happy diagnosing people and prescribing one or more pills or injectables – because there is no money in preventing chronic illnesses, but there is a large amount of money in supplying symptom support for those chronic illnesses.

- Hospitals, which should have some of the highest quality and best foods, promoting unhealthy eating through the sale of sugary drinks and the use of ultra-processed foods for patients.

- Pharmaceutical companies, many with deeply cozy connections with the U.S. Food & Drug Administration (FDA), willingly providing people with a pill for any ailment – regardless of whether those ailments can be reversed through diet – medications that often come with multiple (and dangerous) side effects.

- Media companies (including traditional and social media) happily accepting billions of dollars in advertising revenue from food companies that tell us lies and which are actively making us sicker.

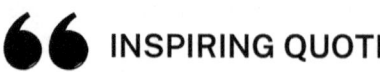

INSPIRING QUOTE

"We are sick. Worldwide, we are struggling with diseases that were once very rare – and in many cases, we're losing the fight." — Benjamin Bikman, Ph.D.

Now you see why there is a desperate need for the Healing Revolution Diet.

FOOD FACT:
Ultra-processed foods are industrially-formulated edible products produced from manufactured ingredients that have been extracted from both real and synthesized foods, processed to remove other items (including fiber), then reassembled to create frozen or shelf-stable, appetizing, and conveniently prepared foods and meals. Experts consider them dangerous and addictive because of the added sugars and chemical additives as well as the removal of fiber, which results in people eating in much larger quantities.

How have we gotten food and nutrition so wrong? Why has the vast majority of food prepared for us become hazardous to our health?

IT'S NOT JUST ABOUT FOOD AND DIET

Yes, many of the processed (and all of the ultra-processed) foods found in grocery stores, convenience stores, and all types of restaurants (though fast foods are the worst) are toxic and/or have toxic ingredients that are slowly killing us, but it's not just the foods that are affecting our health and livelihood.

Besides consuming bad foods, here are other factors leading to our current health and healing crisis:

- Sedentary lifestyle (we should be moving throughout the day, not just on weekends)
- Addictions (fueled by trauma; especially to drugs/alcohol, but also gambling, shopping, porn)
- Separation from nature (artificially living life indoors, separated from nature, foods, gardens)
- Cigarette smoking (because of the harsh chemicals; pure tobacco is not inherently bad)
- Sleep habits (most people do not get enough consistent hours of sleep, key for healing)
- Environmental factors (including air pollution, electromagnetics, and microplastics)
- Culture (a harsher, less forgiving, opinion-based anger; especially social media)

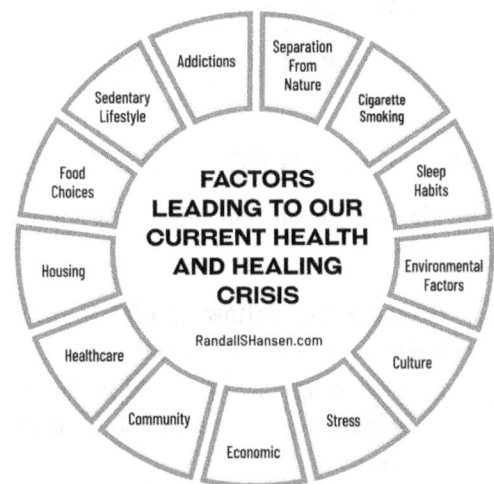

- Stress (increasing and chronic levels of mental tension caused by difficult situations)
- Economic (forcing poor choices in food, hygiene, and other key health factors)
- Community (increasingly isolated lives; current loneliness epidemic)
- Healthcare (which focuses almost entirely on sickcare; prevention is almost nonexistent)
- Housing (real estate and rents sky-high, taking more of household budget; lack of supply)

As you move forward with a health and healing journey, all the issues negatively affecting your health should try to be addressed – but they do NOT need to be addressed all at once, and some are completely out of your control so that the best you can do is mitigate the circumstances.

Please remember this journey is a process, a multitude of small steps to get you to a place of healing and health.

The best place to start – the one item that has the largest impact on our health and longevity – is with the food and what we eat or don't eat and what we should be eating.

The Healing Revolution Diet is about reprioritizing and revaluing food as part of our total household spending. In order for you to heal and have better health, your relationship with food has to change dramatically.

> **HEALING HINT**
> Amazingly, two or more people can eat the exact same foods and have very different reactions in their bodies – all based on the composition and strength of the beneficial bacteria in the gut microbiome. Just one reason why standard restrictive diets do not work for all people.

THE HEALING REVOLUTION DIET

The Healing Revolution Diet is an approach to eating and living based on 10 principles:

1. **Stop dieting, following diet fads.** While diets and food plans have been around for ages, the modern age of dieting started in the early 1900s, but took off in the 1960s – and we have never looked back. We need to stop dieting and focus on developing a healthy relationship with real foods. Diets do not work.

2. **Eliminate refined sugar consumption.** Depending on the source, Americans consume somewhere between 100 and 120 pounds of refined sugar PER YEAR – or about 30 teaspoons (126 grams) of added sugar per day. Sugar is in just about every ultra-processed food, both sweet and savory items, but the worst are the sugar drinks (sodas, coffees, juices, etc.) that some call "diabetes water."

3. **Focus on healthy fats and proteins.** The two most essential macronutrients – elements of food – that people need are good fats and high-quality proteins. The body runs on fats and protein, and yes, there are major differences in the quality of fats and proteins.

4. **Greatly reduce ultra-processed foods, fast foods, and takeout.** The food and restaurant industries have made us lazy, resulting in many more meals prepared outside the home. The majority of foods in the supermarket and in restaurants have been chemically altered so that they are addictive, unfulfilling/leaving you wanting more, and dangerously unhealthy.

5. **Cook more from scratch.** There is nothing healthier or more satisfying than cooking up meals made from real, natural ingredients, including proteins, fats, and vegetables. We need to regain and relearn the value in cooking our own food.

6. **Add more fiber, especially from vegetables and seeds and nuts.** The greatest deficiency missing in almost all meals and snacks is fiber, which is essential for our health; our gut microbiome exists on fiber. The massive drop in fiber in the American diet can be seen in the uptick in gut diseases, including colon cancer.

7. **Eat regeneratively grown foods from local farms and ranches.** The American culture has left the small farmer and rancher in the dust; most of us now buy our meats and produce from the local supermarket or Walmart – meats raised conventionally, dangerously, and inhumanely and fruits and vegetables grown with noxious chemicals. The best and healthiest foods are raised by your small, local farmers and ranchers, but do check that they are following best practices.

8. **Buy organic over conventionally grown foods.** The organic label is not perfect and organic products tend to cost a bit more, but there are multiple advantages of organically-produced foods over conventionally-produced foods.

9. **Grow your own food.** While not always possible, growing at least some of your own food is the best solution for many reasons. Use your yard, a patio or windowsill, or find or help start a community garden.

10. **Improve all aspects of your dieta/lifestyle.** Food is one cornerstone of health and a key modality for healing, but cleaning up your eating and nutrition is just the start of transforming your life for the better. This includes movement, spirituality, nature, and more.

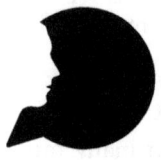

AUTHOR INSIGHT

Even though I felt highly educated in the nutrition space, it was only about five years ago that I discovered the dangers – and lies – about "vegetable" oils; the corn, canola, vegetable, soybean, safflower, and sunflower oils, which flooded the food market when animal fat was wrongly demonized. These oils are industrially produced using chemical bleaches and solvents from subsidized, cheap crops, and meant for use in machinery, not people. Please avoid them as much as possible.

HOW AGRICULTURE AND FOOD PRODUCTION HAVE RADICALLY CHANGED IN THE PAST CENTURY

Quick History Lesson on U.S. Agriculture

The way we grow – and what we grow – has changed dramatically, especially in the last 70 years.

About 100 years ago, the U.S. was recovering from the Dust Bowl, which first exposed the dangers of modern, mechanized farming. The Dust Bowl lasted for almost a decade, exposing poor agricultural practices and bad governmental practices. The resulting wind erosion carried healthy topsoil all across the country. Government subsidies for farming grew at the same time that many people abandoned farming for other occupations.

The 1950s and 1960s brought a revolution in agricultural technology, greatly increasing yields and resulting in more specialized, capital-intensive conventional farms focused purely on yields and profits – many of which focused on monoculture crops.

The late 1950s–1960s also began the chemical revolution in agriculture, with the increasing use of nitrogen to gain higher yields.

Soybean became a major crop during this time, partly because of government subsidies. By the end of the 1960s, soybean oil became the most popular "vegetable" oil.

The 1970s saw a massive push by the U.S. government to encourage farms to switch to monoculture crops (planting entire fields with just one crop), telling farmers to plant as much corn and soybean as they could. This type of farming uses synthetic fertilizers, chemical pesticides and herbicides, and heavy, destructive farm machinery to cultivate vast monocultures of corn, soybean, wheat, cotton, sugar beets.

In the mid-1970s, Archer Daniel Midland (ADM), a big producer of the toxic high fructose corn syrup (HFCS), began petitioning the government to make ethanol, a by-product from the production of HFCS, an additive to gasoline to help end our "energy dependence." From then until this day, massive farming operations are producing huge amounts of subsidized corn for HFCS and ethanol.

Also in the mid-1970s, glyphosate (Roundup), a highly toxic herbicide, was introduced and immediately became popular and put into widespread use for increasing monoculture crop yields.

The 1980s and 1990s saw increased interest in sustainability and the introduction of organic products, as well as the introduction and use of genetically-altered (bioengineered) crops in conventional farming.

The last two decades have seen a further consolidation of conventional farming operations into megafarms focused entirely on profit and yield. At the same time, the regenerative farming movement took hold and organic farming and ranching grew. Regenerative farming focuses on practices that actively improve the health of the soil, as well as supporting the humane treatment of animals.

FOOD FACT:
Americans consumed just above 6 pounds of refined sugar per person per year in the early 1800s; today, that number is estimated to be 100-120 pounds! A simple illustration: In the 1800s, we ate the same amount of added sugar in one 12-ounce can of soda ***every five days,*** while today we eat that much sugar about ***four times a day***.

Quick History Lesson on the U.S. Food Industry

The food system in the U.S. was not ideal a century ago, but most people were healthy, active, and eating higher quality foods than today.

Our food problems started back in the 1950s after then-President Eisenhower suffered a heart attack in office, which sent America into a panic to discover the cause. While many researchers attempted to tackle the question, one researcher, Ancel Keys, had the loudest (and some would say bullying) voice.

Unfortunately, his research was faulty (and perhaps influenced by the sugar lobby). He concluded that fat, especially animal fat, was the cause of heart disease... and the publishing and vehement defending of the research led to devastatingly bad decisions by the U.S. government, health agencies, and the food industry.

Starting in the 1980s and continuing to this day, the food industry reacted to the concept that fat (especially animal fat) is bad for health by reformulating the entire packaged and frozen foods category – replacing beneficial fats with questionable industrial seed oils, increasing the sugar content exponentially, utilizing untested additives and preservatives, and stripping away the fiber... these products, which account for more than two-thirds of a typical grocery store, have since been labeled as ultra-processed foods. Because of the sugar and lack of fiber, these products are addictive and unfulfilling, leaving consumers to eat far more than they should.

Unfortunately for consumers, these food marketers used the mask of "health" to replace high-quality (but expensive) ingredients with cheap, synthetic chemicals that can be combined to create an artificial version of eggs, butter, potatoes, anything – which is why these products are called imposter foods.

During this same time period, farming and ranching changed dramatically too, with most food raised following an industrial model that focuses on moving massive numbers of animals through processing, with a focus on profits, not on health or animal welfare.

Most of the conventional meat for sale in supermarkets comes from cows fattened up in one of many huge feedlots across the country. These cows live in close and disgusting quarters, are fed GMO and pesticide-laden grains that their bodies can't fully digest, and are administered antibiotics for health and bulking up. Similar horrible conditions are used for conventionally raised chickens and pigs.

The same holds true for the fruits and vegetables conventionally grown, which arrive with remnants of the pesticides, herbicides, and other chemicals sprayed on them to maximize crops over people's health and safety.

The foods in today's supermarkets may, on the surface, have some similarities to the foods from 70 years ago, but the content is completely different, having been modified to achieve maximum productivity and to guarantee repeat buyers because of the addictive nature of the foods. Because these products look similar to real products, but are fake and dangerous, they are being referred to as *imposter foods*.

FOOD FACT:

Thanks to the troubled research results from Ancel Keys, the U.S. has spent half a century blaming and avoiding healthy fat, and instead eating excessive amounts of added sugars and lots more simple carbohydrates... ushering in an epidemic of preventable chronic health diseases – and deaths.

NUTRITION AND FOOD MYTHS DEBUNKED

The Healing Revolution Diet is also about correcting nutrition myths and misunderstandings. What follows are 10 of the most heinous myths.

Have you heard any of these nutrition myths?

- Don't eat eggs!
- Cut down on your salt!
- Stop eating beef!
- Eat more breads and pastas!
- Fat makes you fat!
- Snacks are better than big meals!
- Breakfast is the most important meal of the day!

Sadly, it's not enough that our food system is completely broken, but people also have to contend with food, diet, and nutrition myths that will not go away.

1. **Fat is Bad.** Of all elements related to food, fat has been the most misunderstood. Some people still believe that eating fat makes you fat. Wrong. Eating fat does not cause heart disease, if it is the right kind of fat. Beneficial fat is a key macronutrient our bodies need. The fat from pastured, grassfed animals is some of the healthiest and best fat to eat. Sadly, we replaced healthy animal fats with toxic "vegetable" fats in the form of margarine and industrially-produced seed oils, manufactured from corn, soy, rapeseed, cotton, safflower, and sunflower seeds. The other big issue here is we have upset our traditional balance of fatty acids, consuming an extremely high amount of Omega-6 fatty acids, which are inflammatory, compared to Omega-3 fatty acids, which are body-healthy.

2. **Limit Egg Consumption.** In the big cholesterol scare of the 1980s, eggs were demonized – including a cover story in *Time Magazine*. The belief, dating back to faulty research from the 1960s, was that dietary cholesterol contributed to high blood cholesterol levels. But eggs have been redeemed, and for the last 20 years, research has repeatedly shown that at normal intake, dietary cholesterol has very little influence on a person's blood cholesterol levels. Today, after decades of people getting their blood cholesterol levels

checked, improved markers are being developed for detecting cardiovascular issues that may lead to heart attacks. Eggs are a superfood. That said, do not buy eggs from conventional egg-mills; instead, buy organic eggs in the supermarket – or even better, find a local source for farm-fresh eggs from free-ranging chickens.

FOOD FACT:
High-quality eggs (farm-fresh or organic) are now often referred to as "nature's multivitamin" because they contain unique antioxidants and brain nutrients not found in other foods, and which are critical to health.

3. **Meat is Bad.** Meats, especially beef, have been demonized on numerous levels, from the so-called unhealthy fat and cholesterol, to animal cruelty, to the demise of the planet. With this myth, there is some truth; if the statement was that all conventionally raised meats are bad, that would be accurate. Conventionally-raised meats follow an industrial model of production that leads to overcrowded buildings and feedlots, where the animals are fattened up with dangerous feeds and doused in antibiotics. Most of these animals are metabolically sick when slaughtered, so consumers can have plumper chicken breasts and marbled steaks – both signs of obesity in the animals. Animals raised in pastures, especially on regenerative farms that focus on soil and animal health, are healthier and leaner, and because they are only eating their traditional feed, and some of the *best* protein sources.

4. **One Diet Fits All.** The biggest myth of all is that there is one diet that is right for everyone. Currently, the Mediterranean Diet, MIND Diet, DASH Diet, and Planet-First Diet are being touted as the best for healthier living and longevity, often stressing the diet from so-called Blue Zones in which people live longer than the rest of the world. If you want to live your healthiest life, if you want to live to 100, if you want to live your optimal life, then the only real solution to accomplishing these goals is to find the mix of foods – containing protein, fats, and fiber – that make your gut, body, and brain happy. It might be that one of the many diets out there could be a framework that you adjust based on how your body reacts. For some people, the keto diet has been a godsend, while for others, a vegetarian diet is best. The *"no ultra-processed foods diet" is one that should be applied to everyone.*

5. **Breakfast is the Most Important Meal of the Day.** Can you guess who started this mantra that is still being repeated by parents to their children to this day? General Foods, in an attempt to sell more of its Grape Nuts cereal, launched a marketing campaign with the classic and fictional line:

"Nutrition experts say breakfast is the most important meal of the day." This represents one of the biggest problems in the diet and nutrition space: the role of money, marketing, and influence in setting the dietary guidelines and food recommendations. Of the thousands of food brands, the vast majority – including organic brands – are owned by about 10 companies, and these companies spend millions upon millions of dollars on influencing both government and health organizations. Breakfast is just a meal, and many people who practice intermittent fasting often skip breakfast, breaking the fast with lunch.

6. **Eating Snacks Throughout the Day is Better Than Three Heavy Meals.** The thinking was that just like wild animals, we should all be grazers, snacking throughout the day. Sounds nice, right? Snacking all day? There are two main problems with this myth. First, our digestive system uses a lot of energy to break down what we eat, and needs periods of rest (besides when we sleep) so that it is not constantly working. This is why intermittent fasting is highly recommended. Second, the snacks we're eating today are not the snacks of old. Today, the vast majority of our snacks – both sweet and savory – contain high amounts of added sugars, and it has now been proven that added sugar is the cause of weight gain and many other cascading chronic health issues. It's fine to sip water all day long as hydration is essential, but as soon as you make it a soda, juice, or other sugary drink, it becomes an unhealthy snack.

> **HEALING HINT**
>
> The key to your health journey (diet) is to determine what mix of nutritious proteins, beneficial fats, gut-enriching fiber, and healthy carbs your body needs to THRIVE. For some, that may be keto; for others, vegetarianism; for others, carnivore; for others, a unique blend. Again, the key is choosing the foods that result in good things for your body, gut, brain.

7. **Counting Calories is the Key to Dieting, Weight Loss.** Perhaps the biggest fallacy – and the biggest waste of time – is counting calories, measuring all food intake. It's difficult to explain without a lot of science, but please know that all calories are NOT equal, especially in how our bodies use/burn them. Think about 500 calories of broccoli versus 500 calories of pasta. The other problem with counting calories is the restrictive nature of the process, which leaves people feeling deprived, and that feeling crushes all dieting. Stop counting calories and pay much closer attention to the quality of the foods by examining labels for added sugars (the real culprit), dangerous additives, and the use of questionable seed ("vegetable") oils.

8. **Sugar is Healthy in Moderation.** Like many, I try to live much of my life in the middle – in moderation – but not with refined sugar. More than 20 years ago a health researcher wrote that "sugar is the great evil to enter the U.S. household." I quit refined sugars and immediately lost weight, had fewer mood swings, and gained mental clarity. We know even more about the dangers of sugar than we did back then. We now know that sugar is an addictive drug, affecting the same reward center in the brain as cocaine. But that's not the worst of it. Sugar is the lynchpin to falling down the path of chronic diseases, as our bodies have no use for an element in all sugars – fructose – and excess consumption leads to non-alcoholic fatty liver disease. Excess sugar also affects our gut microbiome, allowing yeast overgrowth and a breakdown in our intestinal lining, leading to a condition called Leaky Gut, which then leads to chronic inflammation. Only consume sugar in whole foods, such as fruits, where the fiber in the food counterbalances the sugar.

> **HEALING HINT**
>
> According to a recent meta-analysis, high consumption of added sugar was associated with significantly higher risks of 45 negative health outcomes, including diabetes, gout, obesity, high blood pressure, heart attack, stroke, cancer, asthma, tooth decay, depression and early death. Source: https://www.bmj.com/content/381/bmj-2022-071609

9. **Salt is Bad For You.** After my dad suffered a minor heart attack several decades ago, I remember the doctor convincing my folks to eliminate eggs, switch from butter to margarine, and eliminate all salt. Today, we know all that advice is wrong. Current research shows there is no evidence that cutting salt intake reduces the risk for heart attacks, strokes or death in people with normal or high blood pressure. In fact, researchers are now theorizing that it is the vast increase in sugar intake that has affected salt retention, and that cutting back on refined sugar will naturally lower salt retention that could lead to high blood pressure and other chronic conditions. Please note: added refined sugar consumption is a stronger factor than dietary sodium for the risk of hypertension and cardiovascular disease.

10. **Carbohydrates Are Necessary.** This is a tricky one. I remember when I quit sugar and most carbs, some people told me my brain would shrivel and die, based on the mistaken belief that external sugar sources are needed to keep the brain functioning. Wrong. Researchers have discovered that ketones produced from either dietary fats or triglycerides are an excellent fuel for the brain. But we do need carbs in our diet – not for the carbs – but for the

fiber. All vegetables have some amount of carbs, but these are natural and healthy carbs (as compared to the empty carbs in sodas, white breads, pastas, crackers)… but it's the fiber we desperately need. Veggies like broccoli, carrots, Brussels sprouts, squash, and sweet potatoes are amazing sources of fiber. According to the most recent research, fewer than 1 in 10 U.S. adults consume the daily recommendations for fiber intake.

 INSPIRING QUOTE

"Sugar is the next tobacco, without a doubt, and that industry should be scared. It should be taxed just like tobacco and anything else that can, frankly, destroy lives." — Jamie Oliver

A SHORT HISTORY OF DIETS AND DIETING

Most experts trace the beginning of dieting to an obscure publication – the first "diet" book – that gained some notoriety in England and the U.S. More than a century ago, in 1863, overweight English undertaker William Banting decided to start a low-carb diet to lose weight, which he wrote about it in his booklet "Letter on Corpulence."

In the early part of the 1900s, the focus turned more to wellness (but also included dieting), and all sorts of crazy wellness centers, sanitariums, and spas opened across the country, offering miracle cures, liquid diet, cleanses, mineral water soaks, and other "cutting edge" ideas.

It was not until the 1960s that dieting became part of the mainstream with the introduction of Weight Watchers (WW), which has become one of the most popular diet plans in the country. The basic principle of WW is that for weight loss to occur, a person needs to consume fewer calories than they expend. The problem, as we now know, is that counting calories is useless and time-consuming; calories are NOT equal.

Ketosis came into the mainstream in the 1970s when Dr. Robert Atkins introduced his Atkins' Diet Revolution, which focused on the importance of limiting carbohydrates, especially products made with simple carbohydrates. After being rebranded and separated from the now-deceased Dr. Atkins, many other experts joined the Keto/Low Carb revolution, believing it is the only and best diet.

The 1980s were a time of some bizarre and short-lived fad diets, including the Cabbage Soup Diet, Grapefruit Diet, Cottage Cheese Diet, Beverly Hills Diet, Scarsdale Diet, Jenny Craig Diet, and others.

Unfortunately, the 1980s also saw a massive increase in the low-fat diet movement, forever changing our food system – and changing the diets of most Americans, whether they knew it or not.

In the 1990s, the Mediterranean diet, based on healthy fats such as olive oil and including whole grains, lean meats and fish, and lots of fresh vegetables, became a popular diet – and remains to this day, especially touted by longevity experts who believe it is the "perfect" diet.

More recently, two extremes have become more popular. "Plant-based" is a marketing term used on so many products, trying to attract those who are vegan and vegetarian. Plant-based diets have become popular as healthy diets. On the other side, the carnivore diet (and all its variations), which has gained in popularity over the last several years, focuses on *only* eating healthy meats and fats.

> **HEALING HINT**
>
> Your liver is essential in keeping toxins from building up in the blood, but when the liver isn't working well (perhaps because of all the fructose in the diet), those toxins can be released into the bloodstream and continue into the brain. Liver health is essential.

DON'T OVERLOOK THE ROLE OF OBESOGENS

One other factor that has a role in our current health and obesity crisis is obesogens: endocrine-disrupting chemicals that interfere with metabolism and hormones, potentially increasing risks of obesity, type 2 diabetes, and other diseases.

The endocrine system is basically a messenger system, and when it gets disrupted, the signal becomes corrupted, resulting in things such as interrupting normal metabolism or blocking the use of fat cells for energy.

These chemicals are either used directly on our foods or in the production and storage of food. The most common food obesogens are processed food additives, including preservatives, dyes, emulsifiers, flavor enhancers, and high fructose corn syrup.

Furthermore, there's evidence that these chemicals accumulate in the body over time, so it is extremely important to limit exposure as much as you can.

The exact list of major obesogens includes phthalates, Bisphenol-A (BPA), and PFAS forever chemicals (per-and polyfluoroalkyl). These chemicals are found in a vast number of consumer and industrial products.

Obesogens are also used in these products:

- Pesticides
- Nonstick cookware
- Plastic food containers
- Cleaning supplies
- Personal care items

The key to protecting yourself is to begin the process of limiting your exposure to these chemicals as much as possible. Start with:

- Eating organic foods that are free from chemical pesticides and herbicides.
- Not heating any foods in plastic, including steamer bags. Even storing foods in cheap plastic containers should be avoided; switch to glass or stainless steel.
- Stopping the use of plastic water bottles; use glass or stainless steel.
- Tossing out older pots and pans with nonstick coatings. Use newer, ceramic-coated pans or cast iron or stainless steel pans.
- Using a water filter, especially when on treated water systems. The Berkey is a great water filter system, but even cheaper filter pitchers are better than nothing.
- Going fragrance-free in all cleaning products; ideally, switch out toxic chemical cleaners and detergents for natural ones, such as baking soda and white vinegar.
- Removing plug-in air fresheners, candles, and fabric softeners; use essential oils instead.
- Switching to organic or natural items for all personal care products.
- Limiting the use of flame-retardants and water-repellent products.

You have to take action to reduce your obesogens exposure, as there is little regulation (or interest in further regulation) by the government.

HEALING HINT

In the 1980s, Gerald Reaven of Stanford University School of Medicine made the observation that several disorders were associated with obesity. He called it Syndrome X, which he later determined was insulin resistance. Today, we call this condition Metabolic Syndrome, and it is a key indicator of health.

CANCERS SPECIFICALLY ASSOCIATED WITH EXCESS WEIGHT AND OBESITY

According to the U.S. Centers for Disease Control and Prevention (CDC), here is a list of cancers associated with excess weight:

- Pancreas cancer
- Colon and rectum cancers
- Kidney cancer
- Liver cancer
- Gallbladder cancer
- Thyroid cancer
- Ovary cancer
- Breast cancer (post-menopause)
- Meningioma (brain and spinal cord)
- Endometrium/Uterus cancer
- Multiple myeloma (cancer of the blood)

While not exactly tied just to weight, a study released in 2024 found that obesity and the poor food choices people eat play a role in the increased risk among younger and middle-aged adults, specifically for those born after 1990 – Generation Y and Millennials, but also including Generation Z (though they were not included in the study, but are still eating the horrible foods).

The study, published in the respected *The Lancet Public Health,* examined the records of more than 23.6 million American cancer patients born between 1920 and 1990 and found that 17 cancers were 2-3 times more likely to occur than in previous generations. Translated, it means more and more younger adults are facing cancer diagnoses at much younger ages than their parents.

The 17 cancers include:

- Pancreatic cancer
- Small intestine cancer
- Colorectal cancer
- Ovarian cancer
- Gallbladder and other biliary cancers
- Gastric cardia cancer (stomach lining cancer)
- Anal cancer in men
- Estrogen receptor-positive breast cancer
- Non-cardia gastric cancer
- Kaposi sarcoma in men (blood vessel lining and lymph node cancer)

- Kidney and renal pelvis cancer
- Leukemia
- Liver and intrahepatic bile duct cancer in women
- Myeloma
- Non-HPV-associated oral and pharyngeal cancer in women
- Uterine corpus cancer
- Testicular cancer

Source: https://doi.org/10.1016/S2468-2667(24)00156-7

FOOD FACT:

While the U.S. food guidelines push for Americans to eat more fruits and vegetables, instead of helping farmers grow these food crops, the government subsidizes massive monoculture crops (mostly corn, soybean, and wheat) that get utilized into making diabetes water (sodas, energy drinks, juices), and cheap fast foods, some of the unhealthiest "imposter" foods on the planet.

MOVING FORWARD WITH THE HEALING REVOLUTION DIET

The time is now.

This book and the information in this first chapter should be enough for you to want to reclaim your health. We have been gravely misinformed; some would say we have been blatantly lied to.

The bottom line is that no one – no government and no corporate entity – cares about your health or well-being, regardless of what may be said publicly. Furthermore, please stop listening to the pharmaceutical industry's message of a pill or injectable for every ailment; these medications are barely symptom management, and certainly not a cure.

WE HAVE TO TAKE CONTROL.

Most of the diseases killing us today – including heart attacks, strokes, diabetes, dementia, and cancer – are *preventable.*

With the Healing Revolution Diet approach, we do not need to be on blood pressure medications, cholesterol medications, acid reflux medications, nor insulin, antidepressants, benzodiazepines.

There's no reason people under the age of 70 should be on so many drugs that it raises concerns of polypharmacy – taking five or more medicines.

If you are already on multiple medications for some of these health conditions, following the Healing Revolution Diet should allow you to begin weaning yourself off of most of the pharmaceuticals – with the support of your doctor. (If your current doctor doesn't support nutrition as a way to bring these conditions back to healthy, find a new doctor – ideally an integrative or naturopath.)

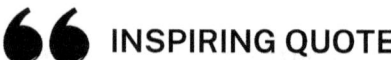 **INSPIRING QUOTE**

"Your diet is a bank account. Good food choices are good investments." — Bethenny Frankel

CHAPTER TWO
The Big Picture: It's Not You, It's the Food

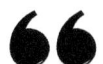 **INSPIRING QUOTE**

"If there's one thing to know about the human body, it's this: the human body has a ringmaster. This ringmaster controls your digestion, your immunity, your brain, your weight, your health, and even your happiness. This ringmaster is the gut." — Nancy Mure

Let's admit we have a weight and obesity crisis. But the crisis is not about why people are overweight nor the massive healthcare costs related to being overweight; the crisis is about our food.

Many people assume if something is sold in a store or restaurant, it must be safe. While the food is "safe" for consumption, it is extremely **unsafe** for your health.

Sadly, this crisis all comes down to money, corporate greed, and the thirst for extreme profits.

Money rules the food industry, and impacts every single decision that eventually trickles down to us as consumers. We suffer with the cheapest, unsafest ingredients in our foods.

The almighty dollar has won out over health; profits are more important than people; big money has influenced – and continues to influence – all aspects of food, from how it is grown to how it is processed to impacting the policies and recommendations from government agencies and nonprofit health agencies.

Every time you buy the conventionally and industrially grown foods and ultra-processed food-like "imposter" products, you are rewarding the greed of massive corporations, and reinforcing that the idea that they can continue to destroy our health, as well as the health of our soil, plants, and animals.

Only a handful of companies manage the majority of agricultural supplies. The same is true for meat processing. In terms of food brands (both regular and organic), the vast majority are owned by about 10-12 conglomerates, including Nestle, PepsiCo, Coca-Cola, Unilever, Tyson Foods, Kraft Heinz, Mars Inc., General Mills, Mondelez International, Conagra Brands, and Campbell Soup Company.

FOOD FACT:

Americans average about 65 grams of fructose per day, almost all of it found in ultra-processed foods, such as fast foods, candies, sodas, breakfast cereals, jams and jellies, sauces and condiments, pastries, breads, fruit and energy drinks, ice creams, and other sweet and savory foods and beverages. Fructose alters the gut microbiota composition and impairs intestinal barrier function through a series of inflammatory reactions. See: https://www.sciencedirect.com/science/article/pii/S2405844023061042

Finally, even government dietary guidelines have been seriously flawed, putting far too much emphasis on carbohydrates, the wrong fats, and demonizing meats. Of course, since the guidelines originated in the U.S. Department of Agriculture, it's not surprising that its focus is on grains, corn, soybeans (all of which are supported with massive financial subsidies), as well as fruits and vegetables.

Why does any of this matter? Because your life and the lives of your loved ones depend on it.

Our current food system is wreaking havoc on our bodies and minds through two main mechanisms:

- The Gut Microbiome
- Mitochondrial Function

AUTHOR INSIGHT

The food system today is full of what I call Imposter Foods because they start with real ingredients but are then chemically manipulated, stripping away critical nutrients while infusing them with dangerous chemical ingredients.

WHAT YOU NEED TO KNOW ABOUT THE GUT MICROBIOME

Almost everyone has experienced a "gut" feeling, right? Well, what if that gut feeling came not from us, but from a collection of trillions of microorganisms that live in our gut, mostly our small intestine? Yes, we live quite comfortably with a whole universe of bacteria, yeast, viruses, and other micro-organisms – and not only in our guts, but in our mouths, on our skin, and possibly even in our brains.

Are you grossed out a bit? I mean, we have been instructed all our lives to avoid bacteria and viruses. And yet, we could not exist without the good bacteria in our guts that aid in digestion, energy production, and the immune system.

The gut microbiome affects the way people store fat, glucose levels in the blood, and how the body responds to hormones that make you feel hungry or satiated. Some even say it plays a crucial role in longevity.

More importantly, the gut microbiome is a MAIN driver in your immune system, metabolism levels, and the ability to absorb nutrients.

We need a healthy and diverse microbiome, yet sadly, over the course of the last several decades, the foods we have been eating – the conventional foods found everywhere – have caused the exact opposite.

On average, our gut microbiome has lost quite a bit of diversity. Furthermore, there's growing evidence that our gut microbiome is unhealthy, leading to a thinning of the gut lining and a condition called Leaky Gut.

Leaky Gut happens when our good bacteria are "starved" for the food they need, which makes them weaker, opening the door for bad bacteria to work on breaking down the protective gut lining. Once that lining becomes thin enough, toxins in your gut can then spill into your bloodstream.

Toxins in your bloodstream lead to an immune response designed to kill/remove the toxins. The problem becomes more serious as more toxins seep into the bloodstream, leading to a condition called chronic inflammation – when the immune response cannot switch off.

HEALING HINT

There are several indicators of chronic inflammation in the body that can analyzed with a blood test. The most common test measures a protein produced by the liver, C-reactive protein (CRP), which rises in response to inflammation.

Symptoms of chronic inflammation include:

- Mental health conditions, such as depression or anxiety
- Constipation, diarrhea, or acid reflux
- Weight loss or weight gain
- Joint or muscle pains
- Persistent fatigue

- Difficulty sleeping
- Skin issues, like rashes or hives

Chronic inflammation, almost all scientific and medical experts agree, is at the core of almost all chronic health conditions that eventually lead to death, including:

- Insulin resistance
- Autoimmune diseases
- Heart disease
- Stroke
- Type 2 diabetes
- Cancer
- Cognitive decline and dementia

The gut microbiome also plays a substantial role in mental health as well. We now know that the vast majority of serotonin is generated not in the brain, but by the microbes in the gut. Serotonin is a neurotransmitter (messenger) that affects a diverse range of brain functions including mood, cognition, reward, learning, and memory. Interestingly, it also affects the body, including sleep, digestion, wound healing, bone health, blood clotting, and sexual desire.

People can take an active role in promoting good gut health with the Healing Revolution Diet, eating foods that are considered either prebiotic or probiotic.

- Prebiotics are high-fiber foods that act as nourishment for the beneficial gut microbes. Think about them as the optimal diet for the good gut bacteria. Best foods include nuts and seeds and most vegetables and fruits (though fruit should be limited because of fructose).
- Probiotics are foods that contain live bacteria, with the goal of adding and improving the number and diversity of the good bacteria. Fermented foods and drinks are the best natural sources.

HEALING HINT

The key to a healthy gut microbiome is diversity. The way to increase the diversity is by eating a variety of different real foods that contain fiber. Fiber is a key ingredient. Another way to increase diversity is by adding probiotic and fermented foods and drinks to your diet.

WHAT YOU NEED TO KNOW ABOUT MITOCHONDRIA

The mitochondria are the powerhouses in all our cells (except red blood cells). They produce a form of energy known as Adenosine triphosphate (ATP), which is the main energy source in our bodies. We would not be alive without them.

Technically, mitochondria are small organelles that exist within cells. We have quadrillions of mitochondria in our bodies; in some cases, there are thousands of mitochondria in a single cell! Besides their main function of supplying power, they are also involved in other tasks, such as signaling between cells and cell death.

We need healthy and happy mitochondria because they convert the food we eat into energy for every function in our bodies and the healthier your mitochondria, the better you'll feel, and the more robust your metabolism will be, and the longer you'll live.

One of the outcomes of the energy production (ATP) is the release of free radicals, which is fine in moderation and when kept in check with antioxidants. (Antioxidants are molecules that combine with free radicals, thus limiting negative outcomes.)

The production of free radicals becomes an issue when there is an excess of them because they damage cell tissue through a process called oxidative stress and cause rampant inflammation, leading then to a cascade of chronic health conditions and damage to organs.

When we eat poor-quality foods – the nutrient-weak ultra-processed foods filled with sugars, white flours, seed oils, and chemical additives – the mitochondria are forced to work extra hard to get the nutrients they need, generating excess free radicals in the process.

Without the healthy proteins, fats, fiber, and phytochemicals from real foods, there is no defense against the mounting number of free radicals in the body.

Weakening mitochondrial functioning leads to mitochondria dysfunction, which is linked to metabolic syndrome, heart disease, and diabetes.

The two biggest boosts to strengthening the mitochondrial functioning are:

- **Diet:** High-quality, diverse, and low-carb real foods. See Chapter 4 for more details.
- **Fasting:** Giving your gut and body a break, such as with intermittent fasting. See Chapter 8.

Other non-food ways to strengthen the mitochondria include:

- Exercise
- Sleep
- Relaxation/meditation
- Sunlight
- Cold/Heat exposure (such as cold plunges)

Boosting mitochondria is life-enhancing and longevity-augmenting!

Symptoms of mitochondria dysfunction include:

- Migraines
- Problems with vision or hearing
- Difficulty swallowing
- Learning disability
- Fatigue
- Heat/cold intolerance
- Liver disease
- Immune system problems
- Heart problems
- Kidney problems
- Neurological problems

FOOD FACT:

Magnesium plays an extremely important role in mitochondrial health and function, with low levels of this key mineral resulting in higher levels of oxidative stress. See Chapter 5 for more details on magnesium and other vital vitamins and minerals the body needs to function at ideal levels.

OUR FOOD CHOICES AFFECT THE GUT MICROBIOME AND OUR MITOCHONDRIA

The choice is clear.

The Standard American Diet (SAD) of highly-processed and overly sugary foods, including most items found in all food stores and restaurants, damages our gut microbiome and mitochondria.

Eating a balanced and diverse diet filled with real foods, made from the best ingredients, will strengthen and enhance your gut microbiome and mitochondria.

In the next two chapters, you will discover the "foods" that must be eliminated from your diet as well as the foods that should be added to your diet – key components of the Healing Revolution Diet.

AUTHOR INSIGHT

You can heal yourself; your body wants healing and health. Stop seeking a magic pill and get to work on changing your lifestyle to bring about health and healing.

YOUR ROLE IN THE BIG PICTURE OF HEALTH

Is food and health a priority for you? Do you understand the deep connection between food and health?

Food companies will only keep producing foods that consumers buy; Walmart will not carry products that are not selling. Thus, all the same crappy, ultra-processed, imposter foods currently on the market will continue selling until we use our power as consumers to STOP buying the crap foods and start investing in and supporting organic and real foods.

To live our healthiest lives, we MUST make food, cooking, and mindful eating a top priority in our lives – more so than cosmetics, clothes, electronics, jewelry, cars, streaming/cable, vacations, etc.

HEALING HINT

Don't rely on your doctor to know anything about nutrition. Dr. Casey Means writes in her book, *Good Energy:* "At Stanford Medical School, I didn't take a single dedicated nutrition course. In fact, 80 percent of medical schools to this day do not require their students to take a nutrition class despite food-driven diseases decimating our population."

A FINAL WORD ON ANTIBIOTICS AND OTHER MEDICATIONS

Antibiotics can be both your friend… and your foe.

How often do you take an antibiotic? Statistics show that 4 out of 5 Americans take at least one antibiotic every year!

Antibiotics were designed to kill bacteria (at a time when we thought all bacteria were bad), and the newest versions of these drugs – often referred to as broad spectrum – not only kill off the bad bacteria, but also kill off too many of the good bacteria, harming our gut microbiome.

Antibiotic-induced gut dysbiosis, an imbalance of gut microorganisms in which the person either has too few good bacteria or too many bad/harmful bacteria, can lead to leaky gut and chronic inflammation.

Common symptoms of gut dysbiosis include gas, abdominal pain, diarrhea, and constipation. Gut dysbiosis may also increase your risk of GI conditions like inflammatory bowel disease (IBD) and irritable bowel syndrome (IBS).

Antibiotics are overly prescribed, often for non-bacterial infections – for which antibiotics do nothing.

According to the U.S. Centers for Disease Control and Prevention (CDC), healthcare professionals prescribed more than 236 million antibiotic prescriptions in 2022 (latest reporting period), the vast majority coming from primary care providers. The highest use of prescriptions is in the southeastern U.S.

Most experts agree that about one-third of all antibiotic prescriptions are not needed, even bordering on medical malpractice – because just one course of antibiotics leads to a profound and rapid reduction of the microbiome's health, numbers, and diversity.

Even more disturbing, researchers have discovered that both antibiotics and many other medications (whether by prescription or over-the-counter) contain "inactive" ingredients that are considered endocrine disrupters, exerting hormone-disrupting agents. Endocrine disrupters are also called obesogens because they can promote weight gain. (See Chapter 1.)

Besides negatively affecting the gut microbiome, overuse of antibiotics has also led to the development of antibiotic resistance, which is when standard antibiotics no longer are effective. Even more powerful antibiotics are being developed to counter this easily avoidable condition.

In the U.S., antibiotic resistance has led to almost 3 million illnesses and about 35,000 deaths a year. In about a quarter of those cases, the infection came from something the individual ***ate***.

Unfortunately, though, it's not just the antibiotics we ingest when we're sick. About 70 percent of all antibiotics produced in the U.S. are used in treating conventional, factory-raised feedlot animals. While other parts of the world have reduced the use of antibiotics in animals, in the U.S., the sale of antibiotics for use with farm animals grew by 12 percent between 2017 and 2022.

 INSPIRING QUOTE

"Our traditional all-American diet is a liver killer. Numerous studies have shown that this diet not only harms the liver; it is a major cause of heart attacks and strokes, the development of atherosclerosis, plays a major role in virtually all of the neurodegenerative diseases, and reaps havoc on the intestines and colon." — Dr. Russell L. Blaylock

The use of antibiotics in factory/conventional ranching has been standard practice since the use of feedlots – technically known as Concentrated Animal Feeding Operations (CAFOs) – in which animals are housed in extremely close and overcrowded conditions. (Read more of the horrors of CAFOs – and why you need to stop buying supermarket "conventionally-raised" meats – in the next chapter.)

But that's not the end of our overuse of antibiotics; antibiotics are also routinely added into the cheap animal feed. Thus, the animals are consuming antibiotics in their feed and given courses of antibiotics – whether the animal is healthy or not.

It's also been researched and proposed that certain herbicides, especially Roundup (glyphosate), have antibiotic characteristics. It's worth noting that all the commodity (monoculture) crops grown – including corn and soy – are heavily doused with Roundup and other chemicals.

You might be – and I hope you are – asking, if we know all these things about antibiotics, why are they so overused? I hope by now, you know the answer… it once again comes down to efficiency, yield, and profits.

Our sickcare system and its connection to Big Pharma means that everyone makes more profits when drugs are prescribed.

Similarly, Big Ag gains huge profits from using antibiotics to increase yields in all conventionally produced meats and produce. A hidden trade secret of antibiotics is that they stimulate growth in animals in a short period of time. Thus, the more antibiotics, the heavier the animal – and all meats are sold by the pound… Heavier animals mean more profits for these corporations – with ZERO regard for your health, or for the health of the animals.

Are all the systems working against our health and healing? Indeed, the vast majority of conventional systems – healthcare, insurance, agriculture, chemical, and food – are all deeply flawed. That said, this is why I wrote this book – and hopefully why you're reading it.

FOOD FACT:

Just because a package of conventional meat claims that the animals were raised with no antibiotics does NOT make it true. Food packaging rules are just another example of the broken food system. This statement typically means that only for a short time before slaughter, the animals received no antibiotics. Another reason why you should be buying organic meats and/or meats from smaller, regenerative farms.

CHAPTER THREE
What "Foods" You Need to Eliminate

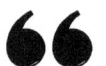 **INSPIRING QUOTE**

"The more we've learned about the dangers of sugar over the years, the more it's clear that it's a toxin, a poison, a killer." — Gary Taubes

You may find the following statement hard to believe. Heck, you might even stop reading this chapter or the rest of the book; but please do **not** stop reading – and please feel free to conduct your own research.

Thousands of food products are dangerous and unsafe for long-term consumption, and they are sold throughout the country in grocery stores, big box stores, convenience stores, fast food restaurants, finer restaurants, takeout, and almost anywhere food is sold.

Unsafe? Hazardous? That's why we have the U.S. Food and Drug Administration and the U.S. Department of Agriculture, right? *Wrong.* While there are many regulations around labeling, nutrition standards, and the like, both of these agencies have long been corrupted by the food industry's big money.

This chapter focuses on the 10 most dangerous-to-your-health ingredients and foods that you should <u>**eliminate**</u> from your diet if you are serious about your health, healing, and longevity.

Because one of these ingredients is also an addictive substance (and perhaps the true "gateway drug" that leads to the use and abuse of much harder drugs), the chapter concludes with suggestions for breaking an addiction to sugar (and the ultra-processed foods that are drenched in sugars).

Without a doubt, most of the foods in your supermarket are hurting your health and certainly your longevity. Furthermore, if you are overweight, there are two triggers in the food that result in people consuming even higher quantities of these damaging, imposter foods.

First, as mentioned throughout this book, food manufacturers overly process their foods to remove the fiber. Fiber is not only essential to your health, but fiber is filling, resulting in a sense of feeling full, satiated. Without the fiber, you literally cannot eat just one serving because your gut says it is still hungry.

Second, food manufacturers have added more sugar to almost all processed foods. A big portion of that sugar comes from high fructose corn syrup (HFCS), which is used as a sweetener because it is extremely cheap – thanks to massive government subsidies for corn. It's estimated that HFCS and other sugars account for close to one-fifth of the total calories Americans consume in their diets. (Soybean oil makes up another huge percentage of all calories; two dangerous substances.)

Within HFCS (and all sugars) is the fructose molecule. High levels of fructose consumption can lead to leptin resistance. Leptin is often referred to as the "satiety hormone," so when there is resistance, it causes us to still feel hungry and eat more of the harmful, imposter foods.

FOOD FACT:

The United States ranks as having the highest average daily sugar consumption per person in the world, consuming more than a quarter-pound of sugar daily, resulting in more than 100+ POUNDS of sugar each year. (Some estimates put the number closer to 150 pounds per person per year.)

THE TEN DANGEROUS FOODS/INGREDIENTS TO ELIMINATE FROM YOUR DIET

If you are truly interested in your health and improving your health, here are the items that should be avoided in any diet:

- **Sugar.** We now know with certainty that consumption of refined sugars leads to metabolic health issues, including being linked to heart disease, diabetes, dementia, and cancers… and the sugar industry has known this since the 1960s. Note that food manufacturers have more than 100 different names for sugar to hide the enormous amounts of sugar used in the foods.

- **"Vegetable" Oils.** These oils now comprise the *highest* percentage of calories most Americans consume. These oils are cheap (partly due to U.S. government subsidies for soybean, corn, peanuts), which is the driving force behind their use in the food industry. These oils were originally designed for manufacturing (back in the early 1900s) and go through a refinement process that includes the use of bleaching and chemical solvents. Labeled the "The Toxic 8," they include soybean (which also is labeled as "vegetable"), canola, cottonseed, corn, safflower, sunflower, peanut, and palm.

- **Refined flours.** Most wheat flours are ultra-refined and bleached (to the point of stripping away most nutrients), and used in baking, cooking, pastas, breads, etc. The health problems stem from the change in the wheat grown in the U.S. to a hybrid focused on yield, not taste; the increased use of pesticides and other chemicals in the farming; and the understanding that simple carbohydrates are unhealthy and drastically increase the risk of many diseases, including obesity, heart disease, and diabetes. These flours are often "enriched" with chemical nutrients to replace the natural nutrients stripped away in the refining process.

- **Trans fats (partially hydrogenated oils).** Artificial trans fats are a form of unsaturated fat that are created when vegetable oils are chemically altered to stay solid at room temperature… and have been shown to increase the risk for heart disease. Food marketers use trans fats because they give foods a much longer shelf life. They can be found in fried foods and in small amounts in some processed, imposter foods.

- **Food additives.** There are thousands of additives – preservatives, emulsifiers, colorings, etc. – that can legally be added to foods without having ever been tested for safety. Not surprisingly (if you understand how money talks), the U.S. Food and Drug Administration (FDA) allows food companies to add new ingredients to the food supply with almost no federal oversight by using the term GRAS for "generally recognized as safe."

- **Conventionally-raised meats.** Just one picture of a feedlot should be enough to convince you to never buy conventionally raised beef. The animals are kept in concentrated areas, fed GMO and chemical-laden feed to fatten them quickly before processing, and given antibiotics and growth hormones. When the cows are processed for meat, they are overly stressed, metabolically unhealthy, and filled with toxins. Cows are meant to forage grasses, not eat cheap, chemically-laced grains.

FOOD FACT:

The U.S. Department of Agriculture has decided that GMO (genetically-modified organisms) and GE (genetically-engineered) foods will now be labeled with the term bioengineered, adding more confusion to consumers who read labels. (GMO became too widely seen as negative, thus the switch.)

AUTHOR INSIGHT
Why do we consume the same bad foods in the best times (when we are celebrating) *and* the worst times (when we are seeking comfort)? Stop associating emotions with food, or, if that's not possible, at least switch to real and healthy foods for these charged emotional moments.

- **Conventionally-raised chicken and eggs.** Chicken is a healthy, lean protein and eggs are a superfood that have endured years of being labeled dangerous due to our misunderstanding of cholesterol. That said, almost all conventionally raised chickens (including egg-layers) are overfed to increase size, fed GMO and chemical-laden feed, and given antibiotics – all the while living indoors in cramped cages and pens. Chickens are omnivores who should be out in pastures, eating grasses and grubs.

- **Conventionally-farmed fruits and vegetables.** The focus of industrial farming over the last century has been on increasing yields at all costs. This philosophy has led to the development of GMO seeds, heavy use of pesticides and herbicides, and depletion of the soil. The fruits and vegetables may look "perfect," but most contain traces of dangerous chemicals, and are lower in nutrients. Finally, many of these foods are practically tasteless; have you eaten a farm-fresh strawberry or tomato? So much tastier than store-bought.

- **Conventionally-farmed seafood.** For decades, the high demand for seafood resulted in overfishing and the depletion of fish in our waters. The result was a movement to farm fish. Farmed fish are raised in massive monocultures – or single species of fish – swimming in tight quarters. Depending on the species of fish, they may be reared within a huge netted system in the ocean or a freshwater pond. In the wild, fish eat whatever is in their environment. With farming, the fish are fed a GMO diet that often includes antibiotics.

- **Artificial sweeteners.** Artificial sweeteners are a type of food additive that provide sweetness without adding sugar or calories. Artificial sugars were created to mimic the flavor of sugar, but are often hundreds of times sweeter than sugar. Not only do these fake sweeteners disrupt the gut microbiome, but many have been linked to a higher risk of cancers, stroke, heart disease, and death. These sweeteners include acesulfame potassium (Ace-K), sucralose, saccharin – under the names of Equal (blue packets), Sweet'N Low (pink packets), and Splenda (yellow packets).

IT'S THE PROCESSING THAT'S LITERALLY KILLING US

Most of the foods we eat get processed – either by us or for us. Cutting an apple into slices is considered processing. There is generally nothing wrong with the simple processing of foods. Processing makes the food more available to consume.

Processing becomes dangerous – and food marketers took it this far starting about 40 years ago – when the ingredients are manipulated in such a way as to strip the nutrients while adding excess sugars and chemicals in a process we now call ultra-processing. Back in the day, it was called "hyperpalatable foods" – because people could not resist eating them… a lot of them.

Ultra-processing adds multiple types and large amounts of sugar, whether the product is sweet or savory. Healthy fats are replaced with mainly soybean oil and other toxic seed oils; this was done at first due to the mistaken idea that animal fats are dangerous, but food marketers embraced the concept because the seed oils are extremely cheap (partly because the "vegetables" used are subsidized by the U.S. government). Then all the fiber is removed, to negate the satiety factor. Fiber fills us, so in order to sell more product, food marketers strip the fiber. Finally, many untested chemical additives and preservatives are added for shelf life, color, taste, texture, etc.

The final result from ultra-processing is a food that seems familiar, but has been altered into something else entirely. For example, McDonald's fries have 19 ingredients. To anyone who has cooked fries at home, it should only be three ingredients: potatoes, oil, and salt; but McDonald's adds 16 additional toxic non-food ingredients.

Don't be fooled with products labeled as "natural." For example, Tyson Foods sold chicken breasts under the "all natural" branding, but a look at the ingredients shows that the breasts have been injected with a solution that contains "natural additives."

FOOD FACT:

Sugar is addictive for a percentage of the population. All sugar consumption causes the release of dopamine, opioids, and other drug-like effects in our brains. Thus, even if you do not have a sugar addiction, the excessive consumption of sugar can lead to the same behaviors seen in drug addictions, including binging, intense cravings, withdrawal, and dependence.

SYMPTOMS OF A SUGAR/FOOD ADDICTION

Not sure you have a sugar/food problem? Do any of these sound familiar to you?

- Hiding your consumption of certain foods
- Cravings that are so strong, you can't deny them
- Repeatedly trying to quit these foods, but always going back
- Feeling guilt after consuming these foods
- Eating in much larger quantities than you want
- Making excuses about the food you "need" to eat
- Denying you have a problem with food/sugar

Can you stop eating these foods? If you can't, you may be addicted to sugar.

FOOD FACT:

"We suggest that sugar, as common as it is, nonetheless meets the criteria for a substance of abuse and may be "addictive" for some individuals when consumed in a "binge-like" manner. This conclusion is reinforced by the changes in limbic system neurochemistry that are similar for the drugs and for sugar." Cite: https://doi.org/10.1016/j.neubiorev.2007.04.019

BREAKING THE SUGAR/FOOD ADDICTION

Let's start with addiction. Is it too strong a word? Only you know. Can you stop? Don't use the word if you don't like it, but please do follow this advice.

Almost all addiction comes from past trauma, but in the case of food, it's also a deeply cultural and accepted practice; almost all our holidays are sugar holidays.

HERE ARE SOME KEY ACTIONS TO TAKE TO BREAK YOUR ADDICTION.

1. Heal Your Trauma. Many people call certain types of foods (usually sugary, decadent ones) "comfort foods." These are foods we seek out for comfort when we have had a long day, been in an argument or personal struggle, or are simply feeling low or sad.

It's the wounds from past trauma that "trigger" us into feeling poorly, negatively. When we heal our past trauma, we break the chains of addiction. Will we never get triggered again? Perhaps, but we learn through the healing process to recognize and respond differently.

Learn about the major categories of true healing in my second book, *HEAL!*... or start with reading a summary of the key healing methods in Chapter 7.

2. Clean Out Your House, Change Your Routines. Even with healing, years of addiction (perhaps your whole life) lead to well-worn thoughts and habits, so it's important to break things up.

The first step is cleaning out your kitchen of all the crap – toss out the cookies, crackers, white flour, sugars, and seed oils. Clean out your refrigerator and freezer of the crappy, ultra-processed foods.

The second step is filling those spaces in your kitchen with healthy alternatives – real foods.

The third step is changing behaviors. For example, when I was deep in my trauma and food addiction, especially when I was triggered, I would drive right by the Popeye's Chicken in my town – and nine times out of ten, I would convince myself to stop and get too much of the horrible food. Once I started on my wellness journey, I changed the route I took home and never ate there again.

3. Discover Healthy Ways To Treat Yourself. We all have bad days, low days; days we need a little something to reward or comfort ourselves. The key is changing from an unhealthy habit to something that is truly good for you.

Discover healthy foods to replace the unhealthy ones. Perhaps a wonderful home-cooked meal or stopping at the local farmers market for inspiration.

A hearty chicken soup or a grilled grassfed steak always raises my spirits; find yours!

Non-food options to indulge in could include a getaway into nature; a cozy, hot bath; visiting with loved ones; picking out a new book; going to the movies; enjoying a massage.

4. Convert a Sweet Tooth Back to Nature. Our tastebuds have been overwhelmed (and changed) by the massive amounts of sugar in ALL of these fake foods. Cutting out sugar doesn't mean we can't have sweet treats; they just need to be *healthy* sweet treats.

But if you are like many who successfully quit the sugar addiction, you will soon have way fewer sugar and sweet food cravings. And when you do have a craving, you have two options.

First, real fruits are fantastic foods – and the natural sugar in the fruits is offset by the fiber in the fruits. Berries, apples, watermelon, and citrus are excellent foods.

Second, there are a small handful of sugar alternatives that are considered safe in normal use: stevia (a natural herb), monk fruit, allulose, erythritol, and xylitol.

Buy or bake tasty items using these sweeteners over sugar and the other "popular" but unhealthy artificial sweeteners.

5. Don't Make Exceptions. These foods are proven to be unhealthy. It makes no sense since they are sold every day everywhere, but the science is clear: you will live an unhealthier and shorter life if you keep consuming these ultra-processed foods.

This means that once you have broken the addiction and made the change to healthier foods, there are no "cheat" days or exceptions.

You may have some awkward moments at parties and catered events when you decline these foods, but these moments can also be a learning experience for others. For example, I had to educate the leaders of a group I volunteer with when they provided extremely unhealthy snacks at meetings.

Remember that the societal norm is the Standard American Diet of sugary, ultra-processed foods, and most events you attend will include these foods. Most restaurants and catering services use these ultra-processed foods and seed oils in their offerings. What I do for longer events – when I know the food will be from the conventional menu – is bring some healthy snacks with me, such as nuts and seeds.

> **HEALING HINT**
> According to Sara Gottfried, MD, the food we consume has the potential to help or hurt first the gut, then the brain, and finally, the rest of the body.

GET HELP IF YOU NEED IT

Please do not let this addiction beat you. It's not about controlling portions or counting calories or starving yourself or hiding food consumption from others or feeling shame over your eating. It's about eliminating dangerous foods from your diet and living a healthier, longer life.

Seek professional help if you can't beat this addiction on your own. There are some wonderful support groups that may be of help, including:

- Sugar & Carb Addicts Anonymous (https://scaa.club/)
- Growing Humankindness (https://growinghumankindness.com/)
- Food Addicts Anonymous (https://faacanhelp.org/)
- Food Addicts in Recovery Anonymous (FA) https://www.foodaddicts.org/

> **HEALING HINT**
>
> Chewing a healthy sugarless gum can be a great way to beat the sugar cravings while also helping with your dental health. I have used the PUR Gum brand for years, but there are many other brands that also use xylitol exclusively as their sweetener, making all of them an exceptional choice for supporting oral health. (Note: xylitol can be hazardous to dogs.)

ALTERNATIVE NAMES FOR SUGAR

The next time you are shopping for food, please start looking at the labels. Food companies MUST list items in the ingredients list in the order from greatest amount to least. (The rest of the food label is useless, and many wish the actual amount was listed next to *each* ingredient.)

Because of this rule, food marketers use different types of sugars – which are all the SAME chemically – to hide the enormous amounts of added sugar in many products.

Here's a partial list of all the names for sugar. The next time you're shopping, look for these sugars:

Agave nectar	Agave syrup	Beet sugar
Blackstrap molasses	Brown rice syrup	Brown sugar
Buttered syrup	Cane juice	Cane juice crystals
Cane sugar	Cane syrup	Coconut sugar
Confectioners' sugar	Corn glucose syrup	Corn syrup
Corn syrup solids	Date sugar/syrup	Dextrin
Dextrose	Evaporated cane juice	Fructose
Fruit juice	Fruit juice concentrate	Glucose
Glucose solids	Golden sugar	Golden syrup
Granular sweetener	Granulated sugar	High fructose corn syrup
Honey	Malt syrup	Maltodextrin
Maltose	Maple sugar	Maple syrup
Molasses	Powdered sugar	Raw sugar
Sucrose	Sugar beet	Turbinado sugar

A FINAL WORD ABOUT CONVENTIONALLY RAISED ANIMALS

There's clear evidence that pasture-raised animals are much healthier than feedlot animals – making them much healthier for us to eat as well. There are stark differences between the nutrition profile of grassfed beef and grain-finished meat. In particular, grass-finished beef contains more nutrients, antioxidants, and healthy fatty acids than conventionally raised beef.

Finally, let's conclude this chapter by looking at a few statistics about the horrors of Concentrated Animal Feeding Operations (CAFOs), which is where almost all conventionally raised animals are sent to fatten up before slaughter, including cows, hogs, and chickens:

- A CAFO can house anywhere from hundreds to millions of animals.
- CAFO animals are confined for at least 45 days or more per year in an area without vegetation.
- CAFOs include open feedlots, as well as massive, windowless buildings where livestock are confined in boxes or stalls.
- The quantity of urine and feces from even the smallest CAFO is equivalent to the urine and feces produced by 16,000 humans. (Source: https://www.sierraclub.org/michigan/why-are-cafos-bad)

The environmental and health concerns *alone* should get these feedlots shut down.

> **HEALING HINT**
> According to Dr. Russell L. Blaylock, in his *The Liver Cure*: "... sugar is not only a major cause of obesity, but also metabolic syndrome, neurodegenerative diseases, reactive hypoglycemia, and contributes to all inflammatory diseases."

CHAPTER FOUR
What Foods You Should Be Eating

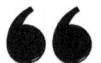 **INSPIRING QUOTE**

"One cannot think well, love well, sleep well, if one has not dined well."
— Virginia Woolf

The Healing Revolution Diet is all about empowering you to consume the best, healthiest, real foods… with most meals made from scratch using real foods.

But it's not just about real foods. It's also about finding the right combination of foods and macronutrients that provide you with optimal health.

 **FOOD FACT:**

According to the wonderful Dr. David Jockers, most of us are consuming too many *antinutrients*, substances that either prevent the absorption of beneficial nutrients in the body – or ones that deplete those beneficial nutrients

WHY WE NEED TO REIMAGINE OUR FOOD PRIORITIES

Ever since the U.S. government and other health agencies got involved in making and promoting food and nutrition, the health of the population has never been worse. We are metabolically sick, poisoning our good gut bacteria (microbiome), while weakening and damaging our mitochondria (the energy source for all our cells).

Because of these poor dietary recommendations and the reformulation of foods that were created based on the faulty nutrition research, we have damaged our immune systems, gained weight, become insulin resistant, and have a whole host of health conditions, such as diabetes, high blood pressure, fatty liver disease, stroke, heart disease, and cancer.

Here are some of the ways our current food choices are affecting us:

- More than 200 million people – about 60 percent of the U.S. – are considered obese… with 10% or 34 million morbidly obese. U.S. obesity rates have tripled over the last 60 years, especially among children.
- Diabetes has increased SIGNIFICANTLY in the last two decades – 38 million (more than 1 in 10) have diabetes – and almost 100 million are prediabetic.
- Nearly half of all adults in the U.S. have hypertension – 120 million people.
- An estimated 60 percent of people in the U.S. have at least one major chronic disease, and 42 percent have 2 or more; more than one in ten (12 percent) have at least 5 chronic illnesses.
- It is predicted that almost two-thirds (61 percent) of adults in the U.S. will have cardiovascular disease by 2050; it is currently the leading cause of death in America.
- The majority of the top 10 leading causes of death in the U.S. are now seen as preventable (through diet and lifestyle) chronic diseases, including heart disease, many cancers, strokes, diabetes, most forms of dementia (including Alzheimer's), liver disease, and kidney disease.
- More than three-quarters (77 percent) of Americans – more than 260 MILLION people – report using drugs/alcohol and/or unhealthy eating/sleeping to cope with mental health issues. (The leading theories target trauma and gut dysfunction as leading causes of most mental health issues.)
- Only 36 percent of people cook at home on a daily basis; younger adults regularly eat out.
- On any given day, nearly 40 percent of Americans eat fast food for at least one meal.
- Only about 5 percent of people in the U.S. meet the recommended daily fiber target of 25 grams for women and 38 grams for men, leading to a population-wide deficiency – what nutritionists call the "fiber gap."
- Chronic illnesses are leading drivers of America's $3.3 trillion annual healthcare costs.

❝ INSPIRING QUOTE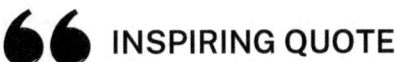

"We live not upon what we eat, but upon what
we digest." — Wilbur Olin Atwater

THE DANGEROUS NUTRITION GUIDANCE FROM THE U.S. GOVERNMENT

The original nutrition guidelines for American citizens came from the U.S. Congress in 1977, via a publication called *Dietary Goals for the U.S.*, which had this ill-conceived advice:

- Increase the consumption of complex carbohydrates and "naturally occurring" sugars from about 28 percent of intake to about **48 percent of energy intake.**
- Reduce overall fat consumption from approximately 40 percent to about 30 percent of energy intake.
- Reduce saturated fat consumption to account for about 10 percent of total energy intake; and balance that with polyunsaturated and monounsaturated fats, which should account for about 10 percent of energy intake each.
- Reduce dietary cholesterol consumption to about 300 milligrams a day.
- Limit the intake of sodium by reducing the intake of salt to about 5 grams a day.

Almost all of these suggestions and recommendations are ***wrong***, especially around carbohydrates, saturated fats, cholesterol, and salt.

Two decades later, in 1992, the U.S. Department of Agriculture (and note it was that department and not the Food and Drug Administration) introduced the first Food Pyramid, a graphic depiction of what Americans should be eating. It included this wrong advice for daily eating:

- 6-11 servings of bread, cereal, rice, pasta (carbohydrates)
- 3-5 servings of vegetables (carbohydrates)
- 2-4 servings of fruit (carbohydrates)
- 2-3 servings of milk, yogurt, cheese (dairy)
- 2-3 servings of meat, poultry, fish, beans, eggs, nuts (protein)
- Sparingly: fats, oils, sweets

In 2010, the USDA launched MyPlate, replacing the Food Pyramid. It was launched with fanfare touting it had been updated with the latest nutritional recommendations. The ridiculous thing is that these dietary recommendations still come from the agency focused on the production and sale of conventionally-grown agricultural products, including many grains the USDA subsidizes with our tax dollars.

MyPlate depicts a dish with four quadrants and a glass, representing five food groups: fruits, vegetables, proteins, grains, and dairy. The focus is on eating low-fat, and extra lean protein sources.

Bizarrely, MyPlate still recommends that about three-quarters of people's foods be high in carbohydrates, including:

- Make half the plate (of every meal) fruits and vegetables; proteins and grains, both about a quarter each for the other half
- Fruit consumption should be about 1.5 to 2.5 cups daily
- Vegetable consumption should be about 2 to 4 cups daily
- Protein consumption, emphasizing lean protein sources, should be about 5 to 7 ounces daily
- Grains consumption should be 5 to 10 ounces daily, with half coming from whole grains
- Dairy (only low-fat or fat-free), one 1-cup serving per meal (3 cups daily)
- Cooking/baking only with what they call healthy "liquid" fats, which are typically unsaturated, including all the toxic seed oils, but recommending against beneficial coconut oil and grassfed butter. *Interestingly,* corn and soybean, the two most popular seed oils, are also the most highly subsidized by the U.S. government.

Happily, the government recommendations also have finally started to come down on sugar, recommending people replace sugar cravings with a piece of fruit and drinking water instead of sodas, juices, and other sugary drinks.

Even with this update, three-quarters of the plate comes directly from conventional agriculture sources.

FOOD FACT:

Conventional farming relies primarily on chemical inputs, including genetically-modified (engineered) seeds, synthetic fertilizers, herbicides, and pesticides. This model emphasizes maximizing profits through high crop yields and operational efficiency and typically follows a monoculture system, where the farm grows only one type of crop (such as soy, corn, wheat) on the same land year after year, aiming to maximize the output from the land.

THE HEALING REVOLUTION FOOD PYRAMID

As mentioned earlier in the book, all the incorrect research from the 1960s is still influencing nutrition and diet advice today – even though countless studies from this century (and in the last decade or so) have clearly shown that we've had nutrition guidelines upside down.

Between the vast amounts of ultra-processed foods, which are extremely unhealthy for us, and the recommendation that three-quarters of our diets should come from carbohydrates (or even more if you add the sugars from the recommended three cups of dairy), it is easy to understand why we have an obesity and metabolic health crisis.

The other problem with our foods is that the vast number of ingredients are produced conventionally, which means taking an efficiency and yield/profit focus over safety and nutrition. Our conventionally grown fruits and vegetables are sprayed with multiple harmful chemicals, including pesticides and synthetic herbicides. Our conventionally raised meats are given growth hormones, antibiotics, and fed high GMO grain diets to fatten before slaughtering.

Thus, the Healing Revolution Food Pyramid focuses on correcting the long-running misguided recommendations while also focusing on the importance of eating safely produced healthy foods.

One Caveat: The Healing Revolution Food Pyramid is an overall recommendation for healthy eating, but as mentioned multiple times already, the key for you is taking these recommendations and modifying them based on how your body reacts. The solution is finding both the healthy foods you enjoy and the best balance of those foods for your health and lifestyle.

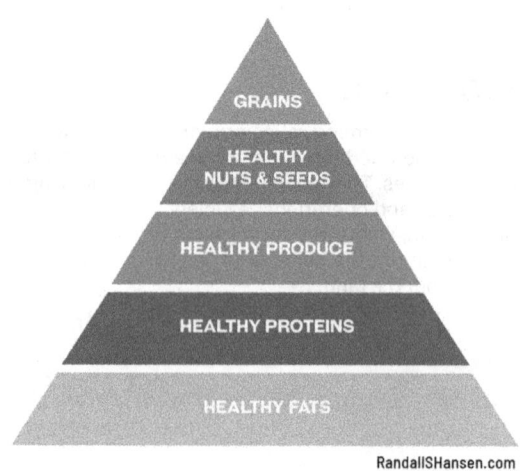

The premise with the Healing Revolution Diet is that our foods should be providing us with maximum nutrients while reducing antinutrients to zero.

The focus here is a bit different than the standard examination of proteins, fats, and carbohydrates – the classic building blocks.

Because we do NOT need to focus on including carbs (since they exist naturally in many foods), the focus here is on these three key nutrients: *fat, protein,* and *fiber.* Underlying these three nutrients is a focus on the importance of prebiotic and probiotic foods.

Here's how foods should be consumed throughout your day, starting with what you should be consuming the most:

- Healthy Fats – 37%
- Healthy Proteins – 30%
- Healthy Produce – 17%
- Healthy Nuts & Seeds -14%
- Grains – 2%

The PURE study, which involved tracking more than 135,000 people across 18 countries and five continents for 7+ years, is a landmark study published just a few years ago; it found that people who consumed higher amounts of fat (about 35 percent of total energy consumed) had a lower risk of death compared to lower fat intake; *key takeaway:* stop eating low and no-fat products. The study also confirmed that a diet high in carbohydrates (more than 60 percent of total energy consumed) is associated with a higher risk of death.

 INSPIRING QUOTE

"Fat plays a big role in brain function, and that's no surprise, as up to 70 percent of the brain is made of fat. The most important fat we can eat for our brains' sake are the omega-3s." — Frank Lipman, MD

BREAKING DOWN THE HEALING REVOLUTION FOOD PYRAMID

Let's take a look at each category of food in the pyramid and explain both why the food is so important and identify the healthiest foods within each category.

HEALTHY FATS

Healthy fats are rich in nutrients and are the *most essential food building block* – even though fat has been demonized since the 1980s. Also, worry less about saturated versus unsaturated fats, as the myth that healthy saturated fat is bad for you has been completely debunked. Just eat lots of healthy fats.

Fats are essential to health and healing, and while many people have heeded the wrong advice of avoiding healthy saturated fats (such as coconut oil and grassfed butter), they are still eating – in record high amounts – unhealthy fats found in the popular cooking and baking oils industrially produced from the seeds of various plants (thus the name seed oils).

Fat does not make you fat. Fat from foods is not stored in the body as fat – but it was an easy lie for convincing people of the evils of fat and the bizarre no-fat and low-fat phenomenon. What *does* make us fat? All the refined sugars we consume excessively throughout the day, every day!

Fats are the best, slowest, and most efficient form of energy for our bodies. Fats are a key component of the cell membranes in every one of our cells, thus making it essential for body growth and development. It is vital for several body processes, from blood clotting and nervous system functioning to reproduction and immune system response.

Fats are also important for the absorption of certain key nutrients, including vitamins A, D, E, and K – all of which play important roles in maintaining healthy bones, teeth, eyes, hair, and skin.

FOOD FACT:
Soybean oil, which is also sold under the name *Vegetable Oil*, has become the LARGEST source of calories for people in the U.S. as the oil is an extremely cheap ingredient (because conventional soybean farming is subsidized by the federal government) and the main source of fat in many ultra-processed foods. Besides the number of dangerous chemicals used to extract, bleach, and clarify the oils, they are also extremely high in inflammatory omega-6 fats, and should be avoided.

The four healthiest fats you should be consuming daily, using in your cooking and baking, include:

- Grassfed, pastured butter (ideally from a trusted local farm or commercial brands from Europe or New Zealand)
- Olive oil (extra-virgin, cold-pressed – and pure)
- Avocado oil
- Coconut oil

You need to eliminate all the seed oils you probably are familiar with, including: soybean, vegetable, canola, corn, cottonseed, safflower, sunflower, peanut, and palm.

> **HEALING HINT**
>
> Variety is the spice of life, as well as something your gut bacteria want. Don't eat the same foods every single day. Mix it up. One of the best ways to do this is to focus first on what naturally grows in your area; next, only buy fresh produce in season.

HEALTHY PROTEINS

The second most important nutrient for health is protein, but the government and health organizations recommendations have gotten this one wrong too, including demonizing red meat, and making protein such a small part of the "healthy" diet.

That said, the key is for each person to find the right amount and type of protein that works for their bodies; just know that protein is an essential building block for the body. Interestingly, another benefit of protein is that it fills us the most; It helps us feel more full and satiated.

Other benefits of protein:

- Helps build and maintain muscles
- Good for bone health
- Boosts metabolism, helping burn more calories
- Can help lower blood pressure
- Speeds injury recovery (because protein is the main building block of tissues and organs)

Our bodies want healthy proteins – of all types. The challenge for all of us is to find both the right types of proteins and eat them in the right amounts. Unfortunately, not all protein is healthy.

If you have ever talked with a vegan or seen pictures of chicken houses or feedlots, you should be aware of how bizarrely far afield conventional ranchers have gone in the raising of animals for human consumption.

All of these animals should be 100 percent raised on pastures. Instead, we put thousands and thousands of chickens into dark, enclosed structures and we send cattle to congested feedlots that are biohazard sites. These animals are fed food that is unhealthy and unnatural for them (GMO-grains such as corn and soy because it's the cheapest). At the same time, these animals are also treated with antibiotics and growth hormones – all to make plumper chicken breasts and more marbled cuts of beef.

That said, the same holds for many ultra-processed forms of protein manufactured for vegans and plant-based enthusiasts. These fake meats are produced using conventionally-raised plant proteins (coated in chemical residues from the farming practices) that are put through several industrial processes, including fracking of nutrients and added chemicals to increase the food's appeal (in terms of color, smell, taste, texture).

Healthy sources of protein include:

- Eggs from pastured, free-ranging hens
- Pastured, grassfed beef
- Wild, free-ranging animals (including elk, bison, deer)
- Pastured, free-ranging chickens and turkeys
- Wild-caught fish (salmon, trout, sardines, mackerel)
- Grassfed dairy
- Organic quinoa
- Organic tofu
- Organic tempeh
- Organic beans and lentils

Buying healthy protein may cost a bit more, but isn't your health worth it?

Plus, if you find a local supplier at a farmers market, then you are also putting money back into the community rather than into the hands of one of the greedy, profit-driven meat producers.

FOOD FACT:

Only a handful of companies supply the majority of the conventional grain-fed beef found in your grocery store. These include Cargill, JBS USA, Tyson Foods, and Marfrig Global Foods SA – and two of those companies are not even U.S.-based. Learn more: https://www.reuters.com/business/how-four-big-companies-control-us-beef-industry-2021-06-17/

HEALTHY PRODUCE

Healthy produce includes both fruits and vegetables, though the emphasis is on vegetables. The main reason for eating these foods is the fiber, although they also include essential vitamins and minerals, as well as flavonoids, which offer excellent antioxidant and anti-inflammatory effects.

Both this and the next level of the pyramid are about the fiber. For the past 40+ years, if you have been following the standard Western diet of fast and ultra-processed imposter foods, your gut has been severely deprived of nutrients, leading to a reduction in the number and breadth of good bacteria.

> **HEALING HINT**
> Fiber is essential to good health. Fiber is essential for the healthy functioning of our gut. Fiber feeds our beneficial bacteria, which results in both growth and diversity. The more beneficial bacteria in our guts, the stronger the protective layer that keeps toxins out of the bloodstream.

Some of you who are following a Keto or Carnivore diet might be squirming with the idea of adding some healthy carbs to your daily routine, but the evidence is clear. Yes, fiber helps against constipation (as does fat), but it's the gut microbiome piece that is essential to living a better, healthier life.

Don't be afraid of most vegetables, but do limit fruit consumption – and only eat whole (skin-on) fruits, with the fiber, which helps offset the added sugar.

Some of my favorite vegetables include: spinach, kale, carrots, broccoli, asparagus, sweet potatoes, garlic, and onions.

Favorite fruits include: avocados, strawberries, raspberries, blueberries, blackberries, watermelons, apples, and pomegranates.

Side note on mushrooms, which are classified as fungi, but most often found in the produce section of the store. Edible mushrooms are an *amazing super food* and should be part of EVERY diet; they contain health-boosting vitamins and minerals, along with protein and fiber, and have proven positive effects for both the health of the body and the brain.

Remember to buy most of your fruits and vegetables locally or organically, as conventional farming uses large amounts of toxic chemicals that leave a residue on the foods. A good rule of thumb to remember: If you are eating the entire fruit or vegetable (berries, spinach, kale), buy organic; if the food has an inedible shell or peel (bananas, avocados, watermelon), you can buy conventional because the peel protects the food inside from the contamination.

> **FOOD FACT:**
> Some experts warn that fruits and vegetables can contain so-called anti-nutrients, such as lectins and oxalates. If you have a sensitivity to these foods – such as joint pain, fatigue, nausea, or vomiting – reduce or remove them from your diet.

HEALTHY NUTS & SEEDS

Healthy nuts and culinary seeds are not only amazing snacks and delicious in certain foods, they are also another excellent source of essential fiber, as well as having other nutritional benefits. (Technically, nuts are seeds, but keeping them separate since most people don't think of nuts as seeds.)

Nuts and seeds have been in the human diet since time immemorial. Just about all our ancestors were hunters and gathers – and nuts and seeds were essential parts of their diets – and yet today, it is estimated that only a third of the population regularly consume nuts.

Nuts have a high fat content, which is of no concern because the evidence is clear that the right fat in nutritious foods is NOT a driver of fat in our bodies. We need to be consuming healthy fats.

Benefits of nuts and seeds include:

- Essential fiber
- Healthy fats
- Nutrients, such as vitamins, magnesium, zinc, phosphorus, copper, manganese, and selenium
- Antioxidants, which help combat oxidative stress and offer strong anti-inflammatory properties

Favorite nuts include macadamia, pecan, almond, pistachio, walnut, cashew.

Favorite seeds include pumpkin, chia, flax, and hemp.

Only buy raw or roasted nuts and avoid any nuts cooked in "vegetable" seed oils and any nuts sweetened with sugars.

Obviously, if you have a nut allergy, get your fiber from other sources.

FOOD FACT:

Consider adding some fermented foods to your diet, as increasing numbers of research studies show the benefits of fermented foods for our gut microbiome. Many such foods contain healthy probiotics, containing live microorganisms that can expand the diversity of our gut microbes and aid in healthy digestion and boosting immunity. Fermented foods include kefir, kimchi, sauerkraut, tempeh, kombucha, and yogurt.

HEALTHY GRAINS

Healthy grains are not a necessary component of your diet, and certainly should not be consumed anywhere near the quantity that the government and other health agencies suggest, but enjoying very small amounts of good grains *occasionally* should be fine for your health.

Healthy grains are whole grains, not refined. In fact, like with nuts and seeds, we have been consuming grains for many thousands of years.

Benefits of healthy grains include:

- Essential fiber
- High in B vitamins, including niacin, thiamine, and folate
- Key minerals, including zinc, iron, magnesium, and manganese
- Antioxidants, which help combat oxidative stress and offer strong anti-inflammatory properties

Unfortunately, some people have issues with grains, including conditions such as a gluten allergy, celiac disease, or gluten sensitivity.

Healthy gluten grains: wheat, rye, barley, spelt, bulgur wheat

Healthy gluten-free grains: buckwheat, sorghum, quinoa, oats, teff, amaranth

TIPS FOR GETTING STARTED ON THE HEALING REVOLUTION DIET

HERE ARE SOME SIMPLE STEPS TO GET STARTED ON THIS APPROACH TODAY:

1. Discontinue counting calories, weighing your foods.
2. Eliminate all "diabetes waters" from your diet, including sodas, fruit juices, energy drinks, and all sugar-sweetened beverages.
3. Break the habit of eating from fast food restaurants.
4. Start making more of your own meals from scratch.
5. Purge your kitchen of all refined sugars, flours, and rice.
6. Switch out any "vegetable" oils with healthy oils and fats.
7. Start reading the ingredients list on the foods you buy and slowly begin changing your buying habits to healthier versions (or start making your own, from scratch).
8. At your own pace, stop buying ultra-processed foods, replacing them with homemade or less processed items.

9. Where possible given your budget, begin investing in more locally grown and/or organic vegetables and fruits.
10. Find a safe and reliable source for healthy eggs and meats to replace conventionally-produced eggs and meats.

FINAL THOUGHTS ON THE HEALING REVOLUTION DIET

The most important piece of advice to take from this chapter is that your diet has to be customized to you and what your body and brain need to function at the healthiest levels. You need to determine the right mix of foods that make you look and feel good and keep you healthy.

No one diet is right. Not keto, carnivore, vegan, or all the others. You can use one or more of these as a starting point, but any diet that has you struggling or cheating is not viable long-term. Plus, many of these diets are not maximizing the nutrients and do not take a balanced approach.

Don't be afraid of eating lots of healthy fats, proteins, and fiber. But do avoid all the ***unhealthy*** fats, proteins, vegetables, fruits, nuts, and grains.

Remember to feed your gut and mitochondria and include both prebiotic and probiotic foods.

Finally, remember to buy the healthiest versions of the foods that work for your health, which typically means locally-grown or store-bought organic.

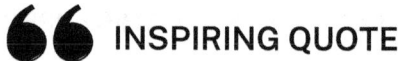 **INSPIRING QUOTE**

"If you focus on health, your weight will take care of itself."
— Giles Yeo, PhD

CHAPTER FIVE
How to Supplement Your Diet With Healthy Support

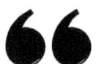 **INSPIRING QUOTE**

"I believe that you can, by taking some simple and inexpensive measures, extend your life and your years of well-being. My most important recommendation is that you take vitamins every day in optimum amounts, to supplement the vitamins you receive in your food." — Linus Pauling

There's a big market for supplements that support health and wellness. The global dietary supplements market size was estimated at $178 billion in 2022, while the U.S. share of the supplements market size was valued at $51 billion. The market is expected to almost double by 2030.

According to a recent study of Americans, about half (52%) of those surveyed said they take at least one dietary supplement; nearly one-third (31%) said they use a multivitamin-mineral supplement.

Supplements have grown from the days of adding a multivitamin to the daily routine to taking multiple vitamins and minerals – to compensate for the loss of them in *all* foods.

Studies have shown that over the past five decades of heavy commercial and conventional farming, the soil has been depleted of numerous key minerals. In the past, most of our nutrients came naturally from plants grown in healthy, dynamic soils. Today that is not the case – except on organic and regenerative farms.

Supplements include products such as vitamins, herbs, minerals, enzymes, amino acids, and botanicals.

Supplements are often recommended for people who have certain health conditions, are at risk of certain conditions, or have a lack of nutrients in their diets. The idea is in the name – these items are meant to supplement a healthy diet, not *replace* one.

Should you be taking supplements? Unless you're growing all your own food or buying all of it from local sources, it is fairly likely you should consider some supplements – simply to make up for the nutrients that have been depleted from the soil from a century of factory/conventional farming. (For more information, see Chapter 2.)

Farming changed dramatically after World War II, so for almost a century, most farming in the U.S. has been conventional farming, focused on efficiency and productivity – not on soil health and seed quality.

All these decades of removing topsoil and not supporting the soil, combined with the heavy use of fertilizers, pesticides, and herbicides, have disrupted soil quality, depleting the soil of vital nutrients.

Unfortunately, organic fruits and vegetables are not much better. They are cleaner and have a higher nutrient yield, but still are not as nutrient-dense as in the past.

FOOD FACT:

"Recent studies of historical nutrient content data for fruits and vegetables spanning 50 to 70 years show apparent median declines of 5% to 40% or more in minerals, vitamins, and protein in groups of foods, especially in vegetables." HortScience, February 2009. https://doi.org/10.21273/HORTSCI.44.1.15

Do supplements work? Can taking one or more capsules of vitamins and minerals advance your health, strengthen your immune system, or improve heart health? The resounding answer is *maybe*. Numerous factors play a role in whether supplements help or are simply a waste of money.

That said, there are also studies clearly showing that anyone eating the current Western (Standard Global Diet?) diet of processed and ultra-processed products and fast foods is not getting the full nutritional benefits, often found lacking in calcium, potassium, magnesium, Vitamin A, Vitamin C, Vitamin E, and fiber.

The debate is whether we can regain these lost nutrients by simply changing diets or whether it's better for people to take supplements. Changing diet away from ultra-processed foods is a MUST, but it is my belief that until we fix the soil (through the work of regenerative farming), some supplements are necessary.

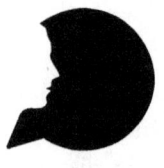

AUTHOR INSIGHT

Please do NOT take any of your supplements in "gummy" form. Almost every single brand I reviewed for this book contained a heavy dose of sugar – and it does not matter whether it is cane sugar, organic sugar, or just sugar; sugar is one of the most toxic ingredients added to foods. The one exception was sweetened with two forms of maltitol, a sugar alcohol.

MAJOR CATEGORIES OF DIETARY SUPPLEMENTS
SIX TYPES OF SUPPLEMENTS ARE THE MOST WIDELY PURCHASED AND CONSUMED.

Multivitamin. These are supplements that contain a mix of different vitamins and minerals. Probably the most common supplement taken with more than half of Americans saying they take one daily. That said, the results of their effectiveness is mixed, with some studies showing better health benefits for women and older adults. It probably makes more sense to determine if you are deficient in key nutrients and supplement directly with them rather than a multivitamin that may contain ingredients you do not need.

Multivitamins come in all shapes and sizes and typically for all classes of people. The key things to look for in a multivitamin include: it has close to 100% of the daily value (DV) of the vitamins and minerals; contains the seal from the United States Pharmacopeia; and has the most commonly deficient elements, including calcium, magnesium, Vitamin D, and potassium.

Probiotic. These supplements include live, "friendly" microorganisms that can help balance the gut and other microbiomes, support digestion, boost the immune system, and improve mental health. People have unknowingly ignored and abused their gut microbiome for decades, damaging their guts with a poor diet, antibiotics use, and moderate alcohol consumption. Some probiotic supplements are also designed for specific health conditions.

When considering a probiotic, the most important thing to consider is the type and amount of bacteria. Start with examining the label, reading all three names (genus, species, and strain) of the bacteria. The most common probiotic bacteria are Lactobacillus and Bifidobacteria. Other common kinds are Saccharomyces, Streptococcus, Enterococcus, Escherichia, and Bacillus. The amount is listed in Colony Forming Units (CFUs). Finally, look at dosage. One other thing to consider with probiotics: some require refrigeration. Note: You can get healthy probiotics from many fermented foods if you prefer not to take a supplement.

> **HEALING HINT**
> No conventional doctor routinely tests for vitamin or mineral deficiencies, so you will have to be proactive and request it above the standard blood test markers in the typical complete blood count (CBC) test.

Magnesium. The vast majority of people are deficient in this critical mineral, which plays an important role in hundreds of metabolic functions within the body and brain. *Every* cell in the body contains magnesium! It is a "helper" mineral that has been shown to improve brain function and mood, sleep, bone and eye health, exercise performance, nervous system regulation, and blood sugar regulation, as well as an effective tool to battle anxiety, muscle cramps, and migraines, as well as lower blood pressure.

Magnesium has very low bioavailability, thus it is paired with another organic compound that makes it easier for the body to absorb. When considering a magnesium supplement, the most absorbed types include magnesium citrate (the most common form found in supplements), glycinate (formed from magnesium and the amino acid glycine), orotate (includes orotic acid, a natural substance involved in your body's construction of genetic material, including DNA), and carbonate (a magnesium salt from carbonic acid, commonly also called magnesite).

Vitamin D3/K2. Humans can produce Vitamin D from exposure to the sun, but because we mostly live and work indoors and the increased use of sunscreens, many people are deficient in it. Vitamin D plays a crucial role in bone and teeth health, blood sugar regulation, immune system function, and overall well-being. It has the potential to reduce cardiovascular risk. Finally, evidence suggests that K2 and D3 may contribute to healthy aging, potentially improving cognitive function.

For the best absorption, the supplement you purchase should include vitamin D3, the natural form of the vitamin, combined with vitamin K2, a nutrient that plays a role in blood clotting, calcium metabolism, and heart health. While the Vitamin D is the most important, the Vitamin K directs the use of Vitamin D, working together to build and maintain strong bones.

FOOD FACT:
The use of statins, drugs that supposedly lower your cholesterol and reduce your risk of heart disease, has almost tripled in the past 15 years, going from 12% of Americans above the age of 40 taking a statin in 2009 to 35% in 2019. Do your research; cholesterol is naturally occurring in our bodies and not the harmful condition we once thought. (See: https://time.com/6287926/cholesterol-myths-debunked/)

Omega-3 Fatty Acid. The Western diet has destroyed the delicate balance of omega fatty acids in our diet, with some studies showing we are consuming 30 times more than in the past of Omega-6 (mostly inflammatory), which is why supplementing with an Omega-3 fatty acid is essential to good health. "Vegetable" seed oils are used in all ultra-processed foods (even some organic foods), and are the number one source of calories of people in the U.S. – and all of them are high in Omega-6. It's imperative for our health to restore the balance between Omega-3 and Omega-6.

The biggest sources of Omega-3 come from the ocean, either in the form of algae or from fish that consume the algae. Since most Americans do not eat enough of these wild caught fish (such as mackerel, herring, sardines, anchovies, salmon), it is best to consider an Omega-3 supplement that contains both EPA and DHA.

Turmeric Curcumin. Turmeric is the spice; curcumin is a powerful polyphenol with anti-inflammatory properties (helping reduce oxidative damage). Turmeric has been used in India for thousands of years as both a spice and medicinal herb. Studied benefits include reducing joint pain, improving memory and focus, contributing to the death of cancerous cells, multiple heart-health benefits, and gallbladder and digestive health aid.

Turmeric and curcumin are fat-soluble, thus the best supplements contain either fat or pepper to be efficiently absorbed by the body. The top brands use BioPerine, a black pepper derivative that enhances the absorption of curcumin by 2,000 percent!

> **HEALING HINT**
>
> If you decide to start or add supplements to your daily routine, here are some of the most trusted and highest quality brands: Nordic Naturals, Thorne, Garden of Life, Pure Encapsulations, Seeking Health, and Zenwise. Do NOT buy your supplements from Walmart or other suppliers of questionable quality, because you'll be wasting your money.

ADAPTOGEN SUPPLEMENTS

There's a special class of herbs ("plant-based extracts") and a few mushrooms that are known as adaptogens, which are excellent for helping the body build metabolic reserves to adapt to the stresses of life. These herbs help bring the body back into homeostasis and appear to help improve physical, emotional, and mental strength and endurance, while also boosting immunity and overall well-being.

NOTE: There are synthetic adaptogens, but why substitute a chemical for a natural plant?

Potential benefits of taking an adaptogen:
- Improve sleep quality
- Boost mood and feelings of well-being
- Support optimal immune function

- Reduce depression and anxiety
- Enrich mental and physical performance
- Support optimal mental clarity
- Enhance energy levels

Favorite adaptogens:

- Ashwagandha – a powerful antioxidant that is beneficial to the cardiovascular, nervous, endocrine, and immune systems.
- Cordyceps – a medicinal mushroom that has been used for centuries to enhance immune function. It also improves oxygen uptake.
- Ginseng – the most common adaptogen; it can be anti-cancer, anti-fatigue, anti-inflammatory, and helpful in both cancer and diabetes treatments.
- Lion's Mane – a medicinal mushroom that may help reverse stress-related changes to neurotransmitters, including dopamine and serotonin.
- Lycium – also known as Gogi, contains anti-inflammatory carotenoids and flavonoids; it supports kidney and liver functions, as well as healthy vision and healthy bowel flora.
- Maca – balances hormone levels, increases stamina and endurance, and improves sexual health; it also boosts energy, mood, mental clarity, and memory.
- Reishi – a medicinal mushroom that helps support the function of the adrenal glands, as well as aid in regulating hormone levels.
- Rhodiola – strengthens the immune system and is used to restore balance in blood sugar and helps with fertility, as well as boosting alertness, lessening fatigue, and combating depression.
- Schisandra – most commonly used as a tonic to protect the liver from toxins; it is also used for respiratory problems and improving vision.

To learn more about these fascinating medicinal mushroom and herb supplements, check out: https://smartadaptogen.com/adaptogens-list/

HEALING HINT

Even consuming the best and highest quality diet does not guarantee you are receiving all the vitamins, minerals, and nutrients you need for optimal health. Augmenting your diet with a few of these supplements may be the key to unlocking your best health.

DR. RANDALL'S PERSONAL LIST OF DIETARY SUPPLEMENTS

Everyone has to decide for themselves about supplements – the value and the type. Some of these are basic and necessary; you may want to get blood-tested on vitamins and minerals or even muscle-tested by a chiropractor.

DR. RANDALL'S DAILY SUPPLEMENTS:

- Zenwise Vegan Omega-3 (EPA and DHA), derived from marine algae
- Seeking Health Optimal Magnesium (containing magnesium malate and magnesium glycinate)
- NutriFlair Mushroom Complex (with 10 medicinal mushroom varieties)
- MoxyVites Liposomal Vitamin C
- Smarter Nutrition Smarter Curcumin (with Organic Black Seed Oil)
- Seeking Health Vitamin D3 & K2
- Osteo Bi-Flex Triple Strength

DR. RANDALL'S ADAPTOGEN STRESS SUPPLEMENTS:

- Gaia Herbs, Ashwagandha Root
- Zazzee Organic Rhodiola

A FINAL WORD ABOUT SUPPLEMENTS

Should you be taking any supplements? Purists say no, because we theoretically should be able to get all the essential vitamins and minerals from the foods we eat – food as medicine – but we know that the soil has been depleted of all these elements because of the heavy toll of conventional farming.

Two ways to think about supplements. One is simply examining how you feel. If you are feeling rundown, have headaches, trouble sleeping, and other nagging issues, you are possibly deficient in one or more key nutrients. The second is ordering bloodwork on your own or via your doctor – but not the standard blood tests, but one focused on vitamins and minerals.

As an aside, most medical experts suggest that people consuming a Western diet need at least an omega-3 and magnesium supplement, but, as always, *do your own research and decide for yourself.*

Finally, if your doctor rejects the idea of supplements and won't even test for deficiencies, it is time to find a new doctor.

CHAPTER SIX
Supporting Health and Longevity: Healthspan

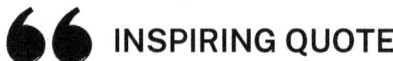 **INSPIRING QUOTE**

"Health is a daily practice, not a 30-day diet." — Unknown

Besides the foods we eat, which is the primary driver for health and longevity, other factors also support health and longevity, and are addressed in this chapter, including:

- Establishing good sleep patterns
- Developing mechanisms for dealing with stress
- Removing toxins from the home
- Fortifying healthy, positive, and loving relationships
- Creating strong boundaries with electronic devices and screens
- Establishing a daily gratitude routine
- Making movement/exercise a daily practice
- Engaging in meaningful work (whether paid or volunteer)
- Practicing forgiveness of yourself and others
- Cultivating a self-care routine/protocol

The other important key to supporting health and longevity is healing your past trauma wounds, which is covered in the next chapter.

This chapter covers the most important elements to supporting your health, including a wrap up of Blue Zones and why it is more important than ever to find the lifestyle that *works for you.*

THE IMPORTANCE OF SLEEP TO HEALTH

Sleep plays a vital role in both physical and mental health; sleep helps the body, gut, and brain recover during the night.

Yet sleep is often neglected... and many people struggle with chronic insomnia, especially older adults and women. A large percentage of people with depression and post-traumatic stress suffer from insomnia.

Experts recommend that adults strive for at least 7-8 hours of each night, but studies show that about a third of us are getting less than 7 hours nightly.

Insufficient sleep has numerous health consequences, including: mental health issues, high blood pressure, heart attacks, obesity, diabetes, dementia, cardiovascular disease, hormone imbalances, and pain.

So many people struggle with getting regular, quality sleep that they seek remedies to fight insomnia. About 10 percent of people take a prescription sleep aid, while 20 percent seek out natural remedies for sleep.

Things you can do to make your sleeping situation better include:

- Use a natural sleep aid (such as cannabis, GABA, passionflower, valerian root, Kava)
- Keeping the bedroom cooler
- Making the room as dark as possible
- Listening to soothing music
- Using aromatherapy (including lavender, damask rose, peppermint, and citrus)
- Visualizing happy people, happy places, happy memories
- Practicing "calming" breathing (such as the "4-7-8" method from Dr. Andrew Weil)
- Praying or meditating before attempting sleep
- Avoiding high-carb and *heavy* foods at dinner/evening meal
- Turning off ALL electronics
- Upgrading your bed, including mattress, pillows

AUTHOR INSIGHT

We not only have to heal ourselves, we have to heal our homes, which often are filled with dangerous chemicals – from air fresheners to paints to laundry detergents. Learn more in my article, Want to Heal? Detox Your Home... and Yourself: https://www.empoweringadvice.com/healing-by-detoxing

THE IMPORTANCE OF SAFELY DEALING WITH STRESS

Stress is a killer. Not all stress; excessive, continual stress is the killer. Stress is also a gut microbiome disrupter, which if chronic, can lead to leaky gut and chronic inflammation – the start of chronic health conditions.

Daily living brings with it the mental and emotional stresses of working, relationships, finances, nagging injuries or illnesses, and more. Healthy levels of stress are good for us – because certain amounts of stress actually improve our efficiency and effectiveness at managing all the people, things, and responsibilities in our lives.

Too much long-term stress, though, and things start quickly unraveling from the stress overload. Signs include irritability, feelings of anger and frustration, headaches, stomach cramps and discomfort, irregular sleep patterns, abnormal weight gain or loss, fatigue, constipation or diarrhea, back pain, shortness of breath, anxiety attacks, and abnormal heart conditions.

Besides implementing some of the following coping mechanisms, it is also important to locate and mitigate the areas in which the stress is negative, overwhelming, painful.

Some stress coping mechanisms:

- Talking it out (with supportive folks in your community/tribe)
- Positive self-talk
- Relaxation techniques
- Laughing, even forced (laughter lightens your mental load)
- Exercise
- Time in nature/park/yard
- Meditation
- Listening to music
- Journaling (using writing to release those pent-up emotions)
- Playing with a pet
- Breathwork/breathing exercises
- Aromatherapy with essential oils
- Gratitude practice
- Setting healthy boundaries

Finally, if you find yourself constantly overwhelmed with stress and unable to deal with things on your own, seek out professional help – starting with your doctor or a visit to your local mental health clinic.

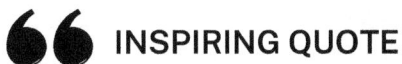 **INSPIRING QUOTE**

"Love one another and help others to rise to the higher levels, simply by pouring out love. Love is infectious and the greatest healing energy." — Sai Baba

THE IMPORTANCE OF REMOVING HOUSEHOLD TOXINS TO HEALTH

We use a lot of chemicals in and outside our homes, and most of them do more harm than good – especially to our health, including adverse health effects such as reproductive and endocrine (hormone balance) toxicity.

One expert states: "The average home contains 500-1,000 chemicals and toxins, most of which you are unable to see, taste, or smell."

Detox the Chemical Use In Your Home. People introduce a LOT of chemicals into their homes; are you one of them?

Eliminate all unnaturally-scented soaps, detergents, fabric softeners, air fresheners, scented candles, and deodorants. If you want some fragrance, use essential oils or live/cut flowers.

Eliminate all caustic chemicals, including: drain cleaners, toilet bowl cleaners, bleach, rat poison. You can clean just as effectively with vinegar, baking soda, and lemon juice.

Dust weekly. The dust in our homes often contains lead, fire retardants, pesticides, and other chemicals. Just remember not to use a chemical dusting product.

Filter tap water. Most city/community water systems process the water, removing hazardous elements while often adding fluoride (in another mistaken government guideline) and other chemical disinfectants (such as chlorine). Buy a quality water filtration system, such as a Berkey filter.

Add healing houseplants. Consider keeping several purifying indoor plants. These include Spider Plants, Snake Plants, Rubber Plants, Elephant Ears, Peace Lilies, Pothos, and English Ivy.

If you have had any water leaks, whether from plumbing or roof/siding issues, or flooding issues, please also check your home for any hidden mold, which can have devastating effects on your health. If you find mold, please get it and yourself professionally evaluated.

Detox the Chemical Use Outside Your Home. Are you one of those folks with luscious lawns, gardens, foliage?

Eliminate all chemicals, including pesticides, fungicides, herbicides, and fertilizers. You can still have a nice lawn (though it seems unnecessary), flowering shrubs, and a happy garden – all without the use of toxic chemicals. Use natural replacements, such as manure for fertilizers.

Eliminate all excess caustic chemicals in your garage: paint thinner, propane tanks, antifreeze, and windshield wiper fluid. Make certain all containers are tightly sealed.

> **HEALING HINT**
>
> Two other potential toxins in your home that need to be monitored. First, are the EMFs from all the smart and wireless devices we own – cell phones, tablets, smart televisions, smart appliances, WiFi, Bluetooth. Second, toxic mold may be hiding behind walls from water leaks.

THE IMPORTANCE OF FORTIFYING HEALTHY, POSITIVE, AND LOVING RELATIONSHIPS

Do you feel loved and supported? If you're like many people, the truthful answer is somewhere between sometimes and not enough. Our modern society has isolated us in homes and apartments, separate from other members of our families, as well as from friends and distant relatives.

Just last year, the U.S. Surgeon General declared that we are living in a "loneliness epidemic," a public health crisis of loneliness, isolation, and lack of connection in our country. In fact, the Surgeon General stated that loneliness is more dangerous than smoking 15 cigarettes a day.

Having a strong support system is vital for our existence and happiness – to our mental and physical health, as well as for a healing journey.

Loneliness is an unpleasant emotional response to perceived isolation – often felt as social pain – and is associated with a perceived lack of connection and intimacy. It is a state of distress or discomfort that results when a person senses a gap between the desire for social connection and the actual experience of it.

Build supportive relationships with some of these well-tested strategies for building real community and making true connections and friendships:

- Volunteer and meet people with similar interests
- Take an in-person workshop, class, or join a group or club (via something like Meetup)
- Attend the openings of cultural events, such as art galleries and music events

- Develop an existing hobby – or start a new one – and find other hobbyists
- Attend spiritual or religious services and be uplifted while meeting others
- Get out in nature and meet people along the trail
- Take your dog to the dog park and mingle with other dog-parents
- Join a gym, take fitness classes, or join a sports teamMeet more of your neighbors
- Strengthen existing relationships that are meaningful, nourishing
- Ask a few close friends for recommendations, introductions to others

FOOD FACT:

Time to stop distracted eating! Too many people eat their meals while using a device, which can lead to feelings of needing more food and has been linked to obesity in adolescents. (According to a study from a few years ago, 88% of respondents reported regularly using their devices when eating; research classified them as "zombie eaters.") The answer is **Mindful Eating**, in which all devices are off and the focus is entirely on the food and enjoying the eating experience.

THE IMPORTANCE OF CREATING STRONG BOUNDARIES WITH ELECTRONIC DEVICES AND SCREENS

Do you spend too much time looking at your devices and screens? If you're like most Americans, the answer is a resounding YES!

A recent Nielsen report shows that adults in the United States devoted about 10 hours and 39 minutes each day to consuming media – including using tablets, smartphones, personal computers, multimedia devices, video games, radios, DVDs, DVRs, and TVs.

We have to rein in screen time.

Too much screen/device time leads to:

- Physical health issues, mainly related to the sedentary state while on screens
- Mental health issues, associated with higher rates of depression and anxiety
- Emotional health issues, such as body issues and comparison syndrome
- Sleep issues, especially when viewing screens/devices right before bed
- Eye issues, including eye strain

For those needing help with screen-time balance guidelines, here are some suggestions from experts:

1. **Take Regular Screen Breaks**. For optimal health benefits, set a timer for an hour, and when the time is up, take at least a five-minute break from the screen. Walk to a window, go to the bathroom, chat with a friend – without screens.

2. **Leave Devices Behind/Undercover.** When going to social events, walking out in nature, visiting people, etc. – leave your device behind... or at least practice NOT using it while doing these things.
3. **Turn Off Most Push Notifications.** Yes, in cases of deadlines or important life events, you may need to keep some notifications on, but you could also change those to badges and not sounds. Otherwise, why are you allowing all these notifications to drive your actions?
4. **Stop Having Meals/Snacks With Your Devices.** When we eat and view our screens, we often don't even remember what we ate and because of that, we often overeat.
5. **Device/Screen Shutdown Before Bed.** All evidence supports NO screens of any kind in your bedrooms. Bedrooms are for sleep and other social activities.

❝ INSPIRING QUOTE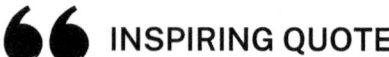

"The weak can never forgive. Forgiveness is the attribute of the strong." — Mahatma Gandhi

THE IMPORTANCE OF PRACTICING FORGIVENESS OF YOURSELF AND OTHERS

One of the most powerful tools for health and healing is forgiveness.

Many of us are actively living with anger and hurt – either for ourselves or for the people who have hurt us. Our egos are "hurt magnets" that like to tightly hold on to anger and resentment – but holding onto that pain and anger hurts *you* more than you realize.

Others are living in denial, believing in our resilience to overcome abuse and trauma, all the while partaking in self-destructive thoughts and behaviors.

Forgiveness is one of those tough ones though, right? We've been wronged, abused, and wounded – so why should we be the ones offering forgiveness? But that's the wrong perspective. The pain of living with unforgiveness can poison your soul and destroy you, so it becomes your only choice.

Forgiveness is a superpower. Don't believe me? It is much easier to wallow in the pain and anger than to summon the courage and determination to forgive... and forgiveness then allows you to focus on other key aspects of a healing journey. Forgiveness can lead to a kind of peace that allows you to focus on yourself – and helps you go on with your life.

Here are the keys to forgiving those who have hurt us (including ourselves):

1. **Forgive For Yourself**. Forgiveness is a gift you are giving to yourself, it's freeing.
2. **Name It, Don't Blame It**. The blame-game is a senseless one; our goal should be to identify it – and release its hold on us.
3. **Take Action to Move On**. Reframe your perspective on everything. Move your thinking from victim to survivor; from helpless to empowered.
4. **Practice Mindfulness/Gratitude**. Changing your focus/perspective from the negative to the positive in your life can help you move forward with forgiveness.
5. **Compassion & Kindness**. Nobody is perfect, and while we like being on our righteous pedestal, it's healthier for us to focus on being compassionate – and forgiving.

The ancient Hawaiians practiced a simple prayer or mantra of forgiveness and self-love. Ho'oponopono is a traditional Hawaiian practice of reconciliation and forgiveness that goes like this: "I'm sorry. Please forgive me. Thank you. I love you." Ho'oponopono roughly translates to *make things right*.

THE IMPORTANCE OF DAILY MOVEMENT/EXERCISE

The best expert advice about movement is that we NEED to find a way to move multiple times a day, every day, rather than one big workout and not moving the rest of the day.

We need to move.

Ideally, every hour, if you work at a desk, get up and walk around; walk a few flights of stairs and do a few isometric exercises. Some of my wonderful health friends and I call these short exercises throughout the day *Exercise Snacks!*

Exercise in all forms induces our whole system to repair itself and keep us in optimal health. Exercise helps us maintain our physical and mental health and increases healing... and yet, when we start talking about exercise, many people turn a deaf ear.

If you're not convinced we should be celebrating moving our bodies, a few new scientific studies should convince you:

- Just adding 10 minutes more per day could save your life. Researchers looked at the activity levels of nearly 5,000 participants ages 40 to 85 and tracked death rates through the end of 2015; they theorize that 110,000 deaths in the U.S. could be prevented annually if adults age 40+ added 10 minutes of daily moderate to vigorous physical activity to their normal routines.

- Longevity researchers found that physical activity later in life shifts internal energy away from processes that can compromise health and toward mechanisms that extend the health of the body. Furthermore, movement and exercise guards against chronic illnesses (such as cardiovascular disease, type 2 diabetes, and some cancers).

- A meta-analysis of 187 studies resulted in researchers concluding that the evidence suggests physical activity/exercise/movement reduces mortality rates and improves quality of life with minimal or no safety concerns.

- According to a report from the Office of Disease Prevention and Health Promotion titled, *Physical Activity Guidelines for Americans,* the benefits from movement include improved brain health and cognitive function, a reduced risk of anxiety and depression, and improved sleep and overall quality of life.

It's recommended that adults get at least 150 minutes of moderate-intensity aerobic activity (anything that gets your heart beating faster) each week – about 20+ minutes a day – but ideally bump that up to 30 minutes a day – and at least 2 days per week of muscle-strengthening "resistance-training" activity (anything that makes your muscles work harder than usual).

HEALING HINT

A good source for an overview on the value of exercise is my article, Is Exercise a Four-Letter Word to You? https://www.empoweringadvice.com/exercise-movement

THE IMPORTANCE OF MEANINGFUL WORK

If you have read any self-help or longevity books, you know that one of the key factors of health, of happiness, of fulfillment, of living a longer/better life is discovering and living your life's purpose. Many experts believe a strong sense of mental well-being that comes from living your purpose also leads to positive physical health benefits.

The Japanese have a word, "ikigai," which refers to something that gives a person a sense of purpose, a reason for living. It's actually a combination of two words, *iki,* meaning "alive" or "life," and, *gai,* meaning "benefit" or "worth."

But it's not just about finding joy or fulfillment in what you do, ikigai is the intersection of four elements:

- Something you love doing;
- Something you're excellent at performing;
- Something that the world needs;
- Something you can be paid for.

The French have the phrase, "raison d'être," which generally translates to the reason, purpose, or justification for someone's life. In other words, it answers the question: *What is your reason for being?*

The idea of finding your purpose also aligns with *eudaimonia*, the ancient Greek sense of a life well-lived, leading to the highest and most lasting form of happiness.

AUTHOR INSIGHT
When the weather cooperates, I love having the windows open and experiencing the breezes and wonderful scents of nature. On other days, I love diffusing one or more essential oils, which are all natural, coming directly from plant materials. My favorite scents include spruce, pine, lilac, orange (or tangerine), lemongrass, and eucalyptus.

THE IMPORTANCE OF ESTABLISHING A DAILY GRATITUDE ROUTINE

Gratitude helps us connect to something larger than ourselves as individuals – whether to other people, nature, the Universe, or the Divine… it can literally change your perception of well-being because being thankful helps break us out and change the focus from (typical) negative thinking.

Gratitude does NOT mean we have to be sunny and rosy and singing all day; gratitude is simply a state of being thankful. In fact, gratitude is derived from the Latin word *gratia,* meaning gratefulness or thankfulness.

Research has demonstrated the neurological benefit people experience from a practice of expressing thanks for our lives, even in times of challenge and change. Expressing gratitude can help improve sleep, enhance mood and immunity, and help decrease depression, anxiety, chronic pain, and disease.

Here are some tips for helping establish a gratitude routine:

- Keep a gratitude journal or gratitude collage, referring to it often
- Mindfulness moments, taking moments throughout the day to focus on gratitude
- Share gratitude with others, showing appreciation for little things others do
- Use your senses, taking time to deeply experience things you love with all your senses

- Change perspective, pushing away negative thoughts and replacing them with something positive
- Do something small for yourself, showing compassion for yourself and your situation
- Perform small acts of kindness to others, such as doing a favor for a friend
- Write a gratitude letter for someone, including writing kudos, letters of recommendation, etc.
- Mindful eating, taking moments while chewing and savoring to be thankful for the food and nourishment

FOOD FACT:
Each year in the U.S., obesity-related conditions cost more than $100 billion in healthcare and other costs and result in many premature deaths.

THE IMPORTANCE OF PRACTICING SELF-CARE

Self-care is a vital practice that involves taking deliberate actions to preserve and enhance your own well-being and happiness. It encompasses caring for various aspects of your life – physical, mental, emotional, and spiritual – to promote overall health and balance.

Three keys of self-care: 1). nutrition – feeding ourselves real and nutritious foods; 2). lifestyle – including exercise and leisure activities; and 3). environmental – how we live, including living conditions, relationships, and social habits.

Self-care is about prioritizing health and healing.

Here are the four dimensions of self-care, with examples:

1. **Physical Health**. Involves taking the time to prioritize physical health by eating better and nutritious foods, focusing on consistently good sleep, practicing breathwork, starting a garden, engaging in relaxing activities, and making movement part of daily routine.

2. **Mental Health**. Involves listening to soothing or uplifting music, working on a hobby, dancing and other fun movement, starting a gratitude journal, reading a book from a favorite author, reading with a child, cuddling with a pet, doing a loving-kindness meditation, and diffusing a favorite essential oil.

3. **Spiritual Health**. Involves activities such as praying, meditating, spending time in nature, attending a religious service, reading/listening to inspirational programs, and partaking in acts of kindness.

4. **Relationships/Community**. Involves spending time with loved ones, building new healthy relationships, accepting help from others, creating healthy boundaries.

 INSPIRING QUOTE

"In ancient China, the Taoists taught that a constant inner smile, a smile to oneself, insured health, happiness and longevity. Why? Smiling to yourself is like basking in love: you become your own best friend. Living with an inner smile is to live in harmony with yourself." — Mantak Chia

WRAPPING IT UP: THE IMPORTANCE OF HEALTHSPAN AND HOW TO ACCOMPLISH IT

Longevity is one thing, but who wants to live a long life with chronic diseases? *Healthspan* is the term: living a full, long, and healthy life.

If you're like most people, you have heard of Blue Zones… places around the world where people seemingly live long lives, reaching 100 easily. But several flaws have emerged from the work Dan Buettner conducted for both his *The Blue Zones* book and all the other *Blue Zone* stuff out there:

- Hundreds of places all over the world exist in which people live long lives; it's not just about the places he handpicked for his book: Okinawa, Japan, Sardinia, Italy, Nicoya, Costa Rica, Ikaria, Greece, and Loma Linda, California.

- An attempt to distill "one way" to live longer; hopefully, from reading this far into the book, you know there is **NO** one method, no "one size fits all" when it comes to nutrition, to living, to health and longevity.

- His plant-based lifestyle overshadowed being a good researcher, and some of his premises about meat are completely wrong, having been disproved long ago, including this one: "meat remained a consistent contributor to heart disease, which isn't that surprising, because it has a high level of saturated fat."

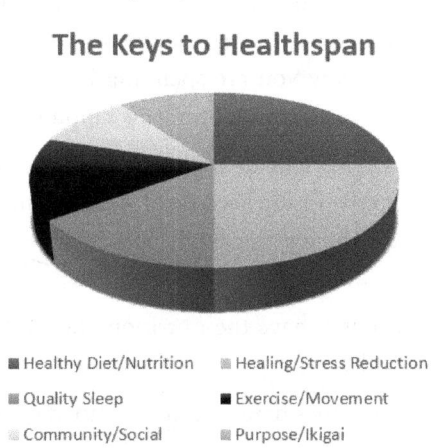

- Longevity is the wrong focus. There's a massive difference between longevity, which is simply living a long life, and healthspan, living a long and healthy life. People can live to be 100, but are they active and happy or facing multiple, crippling health problems?

If you want a long healthspan, here's the rough consensus of what you should be doing. Again, adjust for how these things best work for you – and remember the other topics discussed earlier in this chapter.

- Healthy Diet/Nutrition   25%
- Healing/Stress Reduction   25%
- Quality Sleep   15%
- Exercise/Movement   15%
- Community/Social/Family   10%
- Purpose   10%

The overarching concept is that the best habits for healthspan are holistic, and that your goal should be to keep *building* upon a strong foundation by adding new healthy habits. You do not need to do all the work overnight *and* you can start this work at any age, but the earlier, the better!

The two most important factors related to living a long and healthy life are fixing/improving your diet and working to heal and address/reduce chronic stress.

The food part is covered in detail already, but I cannot emphasize the importance of eliminating those ultra-processed and sugary foods, replacing them with whole, real foods.

I used to think stress was a minor inconvenience to being alive, but the more research into this area, the more stress has shown that it is a killer and debilitator. But it's not just stress alone; you need to heal from past trauma wounds because the energy you are spending internally to ignore the trauma (whether you are consciously aware or not) is sapping away years from your life.

Being in fight or flight mode for continuous periods of time will corrode you from the inside because of the amount of stress hormones released to fight the enemy! The fight or flight response is an ancient survival mechanism driven by the sympathetic nervous system, back when people were in the fight for their lives.

Once you have the nutrition and healing functions accomplished, you are halfway there!

Next comes fixing sleep and moving *every* day.

The final two components are having community and having a purpose, and those two are often intertwined. I know for me, I am often using my purpose to serve and help those folks in my community!

One final note. It is assumed that you have eliminated or mostly eliminated two of the worst habits ever developed – smoking cigarettes and drinking alcohol. Tobacco is not a harmful plant (in fact, in some cultures it is a medicinal plant); it is the amount of chemicals added to cigarettes and vapes that make them hazardous. Studies are mixed on alcohol, but for now, very small doses (such as a drink a day) seem marginally okay.

CHAPTER SEVEN
Wholeistic Healing…
Why and How Health is More Than Just Food

 INSPIRING QUOTE

"A healthy outside starts from the inside." — Robert Urich

Congratulations on making it through the bulk of the book and the formula for having health success. Diet and nutrition are a cornerstone of living your optimal life.

Unfortunately, most of us not only need to go on a health journey, but a healing journey as well. Most of us experience one or more traumatic experiences in our lifetimes, with many of those occurring in childhood.

If you doubt you have ever experienced trauma, please skip ahead to the end of this chapter and take the trauma assessment.

Healing trauma is also part of a health journey because there is evidence that experiencing trauma is a risk factor for developing obesity, diabetes, heart disease, and metabolic syndrome.

Furthermore, other research has shown that childhood trauma, especially, can alter the reward center in the brain, resulting in food-related issues including addiction and eating disorders.

HEALING HINT

Because this is a book about healing, and specifically the role of food on our mental and physical health, Big Chemical has to be noted for its role in the thousands of chemicals that are used in food production and now found in the air and water, in addition to the foods. Fixing our food is vital, but so is cleaning our soil, air, and water.

Past trauma – of all types – stays with us. It is stored as compressed survival energy, until we can find a way of clearing it, not simply masking the symptoms. Untreated trauma leads to a myriad of health and emotional issues, robbing us of joy, love, and intimacy, as well as affecting our immune systems.

To truly heal, we need to understand that past traumas can impact every system within our bodies, and that the ONLY way to heal is to clear that trauma, not simply mask the symptoms. To live our authentic lives – lives filled more with hope and love – we need to HEAL.

Without healing, no one can escape the torture of our psyche's attempt to find fault, raise doubts, question our motivations, challenge our ideas of love and happiness, be our own harshest critic… and even inflict physical pain.

Interestingly, the gut microbiome produces 95 percent of the body's serotonin – a multifaceted neurotransmitter that helps modulate mood, cognition, reward, learning, memory, and numerous physiological processes – which is why healing the gut is so vital. (Historically it was believed that serotonin was mainly in the brain.)

AUTHOR INSIGHT

There has perhaps never been a time before in history when we have experienced a wellness crisis as we are today. Look at these outcomes from trauma and poor diet, all on the rise: depression, anxiety, eating disorders, numbing pill prescriptions, addictions, obesity, diabetes, cancer, heart disease.

HOW DO WE HEAL?

The good news is that a health and healing journey can take place simultaneously – and actually work well together.

When we move from trauma-influenced to healed, we can finally love and accept love (including self-love) – and we know that love is transformative, strengthening our overall health, enhancing immune function, boosting digestion, lowering blood pressure, and improving cholesterol levels.

I am also a big believer in holistic and *wholeistic* healing – meaning I support natural ways to heal the whole person. I am talking WHOLE-self healing, including the mental, physical, and spiritual – as they are so intrinsically connected that we must address the whole system…. the whole YOU. You cannot have true healing, true health and wellness, true authenticity, without healing your entire whole!

As I introduced in the second book in the Wholeistic Healing Trilogy, *HEAL!*, there are multiple methods of true healing – not symptom management with prescription pills and/or self-medicating.

One of those six healing modalities is nutrition, which is covered in detail in this book. The other five modalities to consider for helping you find true and complete healing include: nature, somatics, spirituality, breathwork, and psychedelics.

AUTHOR INSIGHT
When I purchased 40 acres of overgrown forest in the Pacific Northwest, I made the assumption that I was going to spend multiple years bringing the forest back to health; in reality, while I did accomplish my goal, it was the forest that helped HEAL *me*.

NATURE

Without question, spending time in nature is healing. In fact, in my healing journey, nature was my primary healing modality.

We are not meant to spend our entire lives cooped up in homes and offices; we are meant to be outside, enjoying the many benefits, from breathing fresh air, to the beautiful scents, to the gentle sounds, to the powerful life-enhancing chemicals plants release, to the Vitamin D we absorb, to the health benefits and reduced stress.

The Japanese have a term for relaxing in nature – *shinrin-yoku* – which means "forest bathing." It involves opening the senses to the woody aroma of the trees and other plants, the green scenery, and the soothing sounds of streams and waterfalls... because all of these elements play a part in promoting better health and healing.

Simply being in nature induces a state of physiologic relaxation, a true stress-reducer.

More specifically, recent scientific studies have linked time in nature to symptom relief for many health issues – including heart disease, high blood pressure, depression, cancer, anxiety, and attention disorders. Studies also show improvement in cognitive function.

And you don't have to travel miles to your local national forest or wilderness; the research shows it works just as well when you sit on a bench in your neighborhood park – or even your backyard. Spending any time outdoors can help positively impact our health (physical, mental, spiritual), but especially during stressful times – and even simply when taking a break from electronic screens.

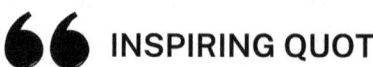

INSPIRING QUOTE
"He who has health, has hope; and he who has hope, has everything."
— Arabian Proverb

> **HEALING HINT**
>
> Research shows that even if the elements of nature are artificial, the images, sounds and smells of nature can have positive health effects. For example, people listening to nature sounds through headphones felt a sense of calm.

SOMATICS/MOVEMENT

There are two key elements within this healing modality – specific body movements to help promote healing and the daily exercise that is important to maintaining good health and to stimulate healing.

Many experts theorize that trauma affects the entire body, not just the mind. Thus, this area of healing operates on the concept that what happens to you in your life is stored not only in your mind, but also in your body – so you need to clear the trauma from your whole system.

Somatic therapy is a holistic psychotherapeutic that incorporates mind-body exercises and other physical techniques to help people become more self-aware of their bodily reactions, thoughts, and feelings. It uses such techniques to support daily functioning and overall mental healing.

The idea behind somatic therapy is that it helps release the repressed tension/trauma that negatively affects your physical and emotional well-being. Healers use both psychotherapy and physical therapy approaches to help release those built-up tensions that are negatively affecting our physical and emotional well-being.

Multiple methods exist for physically releasing trauma, including: laughing, tapping, dancing, shaking, bodywork/massage therapy, walking, chakra balancing, sound therapy, yoga, somatics, exercise therapy, grounding, and Reiki.

Researchers have discovered regular exercise may be more effective than medication for the treatment of mental illness, as well as improve overall wellness. Published in the *British Journal of Sports Medicine*, the study is one of the most extensive pieces of research to date – and based on their findings, the study concludes that exercise reduced symptoms of depression and anxiety.

> **HEALING HINT**
>
> In 2019 more, than 64 million Americans had a gym membership – about 20 percent of the population. But remember, a gym membership is NOT required to get exercise.

SPIRITUALITY

Without question, "we are spiritual beings – having a human experience," per the powerful words from the French philosopher, Pierre Teilhard de Chardin.

Spirituality practice includes prayer, meditation, mindfulness, and affirmations.

Spirituality can be a positive force for healing, especially now when so many of us feel disconnected from the people and world around us. More than 3,000 studies indicate that religion and spirituality have a potentially beneficial effect on health, and health is a vital part of healing.

Spirituality simply means having a connection to something bigger than ourselves (aka, "a higher power"), and it typically involves a search for an understanding of our place in the universe. People may describe a spiritual experience as sacred or transcendent... or simply a deep sense of aliveness and interconnectedness. Spirituality practices often result in positive emotions, such as peace, awe, contentment, gratitude, and acceptance.

Spiritual healing is the practice (and experience) of trying to rebuild that connection – about restoring, harmonizing, and balancing our spirit/soul. For those who never had much of a spiritual life, spiritual healing can lead to a great spiritual awakening.

Finally, spirituality also is about the invisible energy flowing within us; when that energy becomes disrupted from trauma, illnesses ensue. While some people believe this energy comes from a higher power or deity, others believe it originates from within ourselves, but you should know that everything in the universe consists of energy.

Because the focus is on spirituality – in all its forms – rather than organized religion, it opens us up to numerous avenues for healing, including prayer, meditation, mindfulness. From research, we know these actions can result in reducing our heart rate, lowering blood pressure, decreasing respiration, reducing perspiration, decreasing stress hormones... and increasing anti-aging hormones.

According to researchers Matt Snapp and Lisa Hare, there is substantial evidence that spiritual well-being is an important determinant of overall health, longevity, and quality of life. (See: https://pubmed.ncbi.nlm.nih.gov/33513580/)

 INSPIRING QUOTE

"Any time we feel spiritually empty, whether through sadness, depression, or boredom, it's easy to reach for food to fill that void. Soon, we mistake spiritual hunger for physical hunger, and food becomes the immediate answer to any drop in well-being." — Joyce Meyer

BREATHWORK

There's transformative power in performing various breathing exercises, including the ability to alter your consciousness for healing. People often perform breathwork to improve mental, physical, and spiritual well-being.

Many people find the idea of breathwork odd, since breathing is one of those automatic functions (along with our heartbeat and digestion). Breathing is handled by a subconscious part of the brain called the medulla, which automatically controls breathing as well as heart rate and blood pressure.

At its core, breathwork is about taking control of our breathing, and is designed to bring a focus to our breathing, helping to calm our stress levels, lower blood pressure, and bring balance to our bodies.

Breathwork practices have been used by people for thousands of years, and it has roots in yoga. The basic idea of breathwork is to release toxins and stress when you breathe out and nourish your mind and body when you breathe in.

By simply focusing on your breathing, you can help elevate your mood while lowering inflammation levels… all on your way to healing or to help maintain your health and healing.

By incorporating breathing exercises into your daily routine, you may be able to get rid of several pills and supplements you're currently taking, including antidepressants, anxiolytics, painkillers, statins, antacids, sleeping pills, and many more.

The good news is that you don't need any equipment or special props or tools to start a breathwork practice. And, at least in the beginning (and depending on your goals), doing breathwork may only take 5 minutes out of your day. As you go deeper, your time spent with breathwork will likely increase.

> **HEALING HINT**
> In the yoga tradition, the breath is said to carry a person's life force. The breath is considered a conduit of life. It is the physical manifestation of your chi – or lifeforce energy – and you do it 23,000 times a day.

PSYCHEDELICS

These substances are perhaps the greatest advancement in healing in modern times, though indigenous and native cultures have been using psychedelic plants and fungi for thousands of years. While you may be vaguely aware of psychedelics (and especially LSD) from the War on Drugs and the incredible amount of lies and propaganda, I can assure you these substances are indeed medicines for TRUE healing.

Psychedelics are a classification of substances that include plants and chemical compounds that produce unique experiences that can result in true healing, *getting to the root cause of trauma,* and helping the journeyer understand the nature of the trauma and how to recover from it.

As I discussed in detail in my first book in the Wholeistic Healing Trilogy, *Triumph Over Trauma*, these psychedelic compounds are being labeled "breakthrough" medicines, even though they have been around for centuries. In fact, psychedelics were being researched and touted as miracle drugs back in the 1960s – when many therapists used psychedelics as a tool in therapy.

FOOD FACT:
While psychedelic substances, some of the safest on the planet, are illegal, it is interesting to note that two of the most abused drugs – alcohol and tobacco/nicotine – are legal. (And the absolutely worst "legal" drug still on the market for people of ALL ages? **Sugar**.)

Traditional psychedelics, including LSD, psilocybin, mescaline, and DMT, affect the brain's serotonin system, primarily by binding to the serotonin 2A (5HT-2A) receptor. Other substances with known hallucinogenic properties (such as ketamine, MDMA, and other compounds) have different targets in the brain but still produce some psychedelic effects.

Based on anecdotal data, psychedelics are some of the fastest ways to obtain true healing. Many people report that one psychedelic experience is tantamount to 7 years of talk-therapy… and just about everyone who has undergone a psychedelic journey describes it as one of the most profound experiences of their lives.

That said, consuming psychedelics without completing the integration of your journey into your regular life is like going to an expert for advice and then completely ignoring that advice. One of the biggest misunderstandings of psychedelics is that they are a cure-all… that they are miracle medicines.

HEALING HINT
We used to believe that the brain peaks in your twenties and starts heading downhill after age 26. Now, however, with new research and understanding, we know that with the right lifestyle and holistic healing, as well as with the use of psychedelic plant medicines, you can keep strengthening and growing your brain (neuroplasticity) regardless of age.

Psychedelics are miraculous, but not magical by themselves. Psychedelics have proven power to change the brain and help people with numerous mental conditions, but their power comes from being a *tool users can employ to heal themselves.* **YOU** are responsible for doing the work!

TRAUMA ASSESSMENT

Directions: Answer yes or no to the following statements.

WARNING: Some of these statements may be triggering to you.

Have you ever had frequent thoughts like…

1. I hate myself;
2. I feel broken inside, like something is missing;
3. I know I am not living my best life;
4. I just do not know what is wrong with me;
5. I spend too much time rehashing/living in the past;
6. I keep waiting for and expecting my best life;
7. I can't function well on many days;
8. I can't seem to find my true love, any love;
9. I have unexplainable chronic pain;
10. I don't know why many others are succeeding much more than me;
11. I spend too many days drinking away my troubles;
12. I am tired of battling depression, anxiety;
13. I engage in risky behavior to prove I'm alive;
14. I wear many masks to hide my true self;
15. I often feel disconnected from the world;
16. I am hurting and just not sure how much more I can take.

SCORING: The point of this exercise is for you to go inward, both for responding to these statements as honestly as possible, but also to help start the process of self-discovery of past trauma wounds – wounds that need healing.

One of the greatest things you can do for yourself is release the hold that past trauma wounds have on your body, spirit, mind. A healing journey takes you to places in which you can find healing, find closure, find forgiveness, find love, find peace.

A FINAL WORD ABOUT HEALING

Working on improving your health without also taking on your past trauma would be like planting a garden but never watering or tending to it… the planting was a great start, but in order to get the fruits and veggies, *there is more work to be done.*

Fixing our food, nutrition, and health is fantastic, especially for our children. But if after we fix our food and our guts we still have moments of anxiety, fear, anger, aggression, then to obtain that long healthspan, we need to heal our wounds from past trauma.

That's why I recommend, if you can, to do both a health and healing journey; they work well together in bringing health, peace, love, joy.

Facing our past can be scary, intimidating, but necessary. We are not WHOLE, not our true selves, until we find healing.

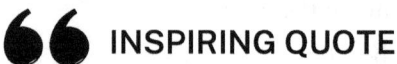 **INSPIRING QUOTE**

"Today's children are MORE at risk from poor nutrition than they are from drugs, alcohol, and tobacco COMBINED." — Dr. David Katz

CHAPTER EIGHT
Health, Nutrition, and Diet FAQs

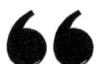 **INSPIRING QUOTE**

"We struggle with eating healthily, obesity, and access to good nutrition for everyone. But we have a great opportunity to get on the right side of this battle by beginning to think differently about the way that we eat and the way that we approach food." — Marcus Samuelsson

Let's clear up a lot of questions and confusion about food, nutrition, and diets.

Of all the topics that can have an impact on our health, healing, and longevity, nutrition is the one that has seen the most controversy, leading to a large number of questions. Many of these issues have been addressed earlier in the book, but they are presented here for quick access to the answers to your questions.

But before jumping into these questions and answers, let's define health, healing, and longevity.

Health: The absence of disease/illness while living in a state of physical, mental, emotional, and social homeostasis and well-being. A healthy lifestyle helps lead to a full life, lived with happiness and positivity.

Healing: A process of acknowledgment, acceptance, forgiveness, and integration of the emotional wounds from painful life experiences/traumas. A healing journey is the exploration and reconciliation of one's entire life.

Longevity: Living longer than others. The word comes from the Latin word *longaevitās*, including the roots *longus* (long) and *aevum* (age), which combine into a concept that means living a long life... living a greater duration of life. (What we should be talking about is healthspan, a healthy lifespan.)

> 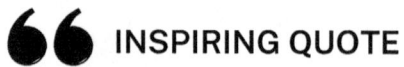 **INSPIRING QUOTE**
>
> "...diets make you feel hungry, grumpy, agitated, irritated, and deprived."
> — Kate Deering

HEALTH, NUTRITION, AND DIET FAQS

This chapter answers the 35 most frequently asked questions about nutrition.

1. What's the best diet to follow – to lose weight? For longevity?

There is no one best diet for everyone. The nonsense you read and hear about diets and dieting, and that one diet is better than all others is simply noise… noise you need to avoid.

The best diet you should follow is the one that you create for yourself – and that works for you. Now, this does not mean you should go on a milkshake diet because you love milkshakes. But it does mean piecing together the healthy foods and drinks – separate from any one diet – to produce your meals.

Let me give you an example. A dear friend of mine suffered with undiagnosed Lyme Disease for decades. When she was finally diagnosed, she was told to go on a vegan diet to help her heal. She ended up losing weight, getting sicker. Through a stroke of God, someone suggested she try the carnivore diet. Her health immediately improved and she started gaining weight. For her, an all-meat diet works – and works well – but I wouldn't recommend that diet for everyone.

Here's what must be in whatever diet you decide upon.

First, change your thinking from diet to lifestyle because a diet is often perceived as restrictive, which is why most diets never work. You should not need "cheat" days or "bonus" days that allow you to eat whatever you want. Instead, you should be creating a diet/lifestyle that does NOT seem restrictive. For many, the one sticking point is sugar, which has been proven to be a drug with addictive properties – and there are many of us who are either addicted or have made sugar an integral part of our lives. Look at every major holiday – they are all sugar holidays now.

Second, your diet must include elements the body and brain need for functioning, which means it must include healthy proteins and fats. There's not much need for carbohydrates, especially simple carbs. We used to think carbs were necessary for body/brain function, but healthy fats can just as easily be converted to energy as carbs. That said, healthy and complex carbs are a good thing – especially those found in vegetables and nuts. The final element has to be fiber. Most of us don't get enough fiber, which is especially true for those who eat packaged foods and fast foods.

Third, if this strategy is too broad for you, then take a look at all the mainstream diets – keto, paleo, carnivore, vegetarian, vegan, and Mediterranean – and try one that seems to most resonate with you, and keep trying until you find one that works best, even if you have to modify it to fit your life. Remember that the best diets are ones in which you feel your best – mentally and physically.

> **HEALING HINT**
> Dietary fiber is a super-nutrient, especially for your gut microbiome. People eating healthy fiber have a reduced risk of heart attacks, strokes, high cholesterol, obesity, type 2 diabetes, and some cancers.

2. What's the best balance of carbs, fat, and protein in my diet?

Unfortunately, there is no magic formula for the perfect balance of nutrients. Everyone needs to find the balance that works for them, but the Healing Revolution Food Pyramid discussed in Chapter 4 is a good starting point.

How do you know what combination of foods works best for you? Your body and brain will tell you! If you are gaining weight, feeling sluggish, having physical/emotional highs and lows, experiencing brain fog, and other negative experiences, then the foods you are eating are not serving you.

To find that ideal balance, you must start preparing your meals from scratch so you can avoid all the unnecessary ingredients that are added to most prepared foods and meals – and so you can source the highest quality ingredients you can afford.

The quality of the foods is an important consideration. We have a conventional food system that overuses chemicals (fertilizers, pesticides, herbicides) that transfer directly into our bodies and bloodstreams. Whatever foods you choose to eat must be of the highest quality – which means buying local or organic.

Here's what I can tell you. Our bodies need protein and fat. Our bodies do not need carbs, but they do need fiber – and often that fiber comes from foods that have carbs. That said, carbs are not the enemy here; it's the type of carbs, how often we're consuming them, and why we're eating them that matters.

My one concern with vegetarian and vegan diets is obtaining enough fat and protein… but as long as you have quality sources of these, and if a plant-based diet works for you, go for it.

3. Isn't fat bad for you, especially your heart?

One of the biggest misconceptions/lies we have been told for decades now is that fat is evil and that fat causes/enhances cardiovascular disease. Completely wrong, but it is so ingrained in our culture that some dietitians and nutritionists still advise their clients to avoid fats, especially animal fats.

The problem boils down to bad research from the 1950s and 1960s. A researcher named Ancel Keys studied populations from around the world and concluded that fat was the cause of cardiovascular disease and thus, if we wanted to reduce the risk of heart attacks, we needed to eliminate fat from our diets. The trouble arose because he was predisposed to this conclusion and researchers returning to his original data clearly found that it was *refined/processed sugars* that are primarily correlated with heart disease, *not fats*.

Because of this faulty research, we went down a rabbit hole of demonizing healthy fats (such as found in butter from grassfed cows) to creating margarine and other unhealthy fats, including toxic seed ("vegetable") oils. Food marketers jumped on "low-fat" and "no-fat" versions of their products, which often substituted more sugar and chemicals for the fats.

With that said, not all fats are equal. Please worry less about saturated fats versus unsaturated fats, but do concern yourself with the ratio of omega-3 "fats" and omega-6 "fats." Researchers say omega-6s are pro-inflammatory, while omega-3s are anti-inflammatory. We need both types of fats, but because of the reaction to the faulty research results, much of our good and healthy fats have been replaced, and most of us have a very unbalanced ratio of omega-3 to omega-6 fats.

Unfortunately, our Western diets (which are loaded with omega-6 seed oils) have an omega-6 to omega-3 ratio that is much higher than is ideal for our bodies – and extremely higher than our ancestors. Most likely you will need to enhance your omega-3 consumption by eating more fish or grassfed beef and/or taking an omega-3 supplement.

My favorite fats? Butter (only organic and/or grassfed), avocado oil, olive oil, and coconut oil. (I don't consume it, but rendered lard from pastured animals is also a good fat.)

HEALING HINT

Seeking healthy fat in your diet? Consider eating pastured, grassfed beef; grassfed butter; fatty fish (especially trout and salmon); nuts and seeds; avocados; MCT/coconut oil; extra-virgin olive oil; quality cheese; and whole eggs.

AUTHOR INSIGHT

Read all the details about sugar in my article, The Deadly Truth About Our Sugar Addiction: https://www.empoweringadvice.com/deadly-truth-about-sugar-addiction

4. Sugars are carbs, which are needed, right? How bad is sugar – really?

I'm not going to sugarcoat this (pun intended): refined sugar is a poisonous, addictive drug that has crept into every aspect of our food production. *Sugar is insidious.*

Interestingly, the body has ZERO need for any refined sugar. Sugar has zero use in the body, and in fact is a dangerous toxin for the liver. Do not confuse internal blood sugar (called glucose), which the body manufactures, with external sugar sources.

Sugar can be found not only in sodas, energy drinks, and sweet cookies, donuts, and cakes, but also in frozen pizzas, crackers, breads, pastas, sauces, and condiments.

It's also in almost every item on the menu of every type of restaurant and takeout food joint.

On average, people eating Western diets (also called the Standard American Diet) consume about 100-120 pounds of sugar per year – about 30 teaspoons a DAY – because of how prevalent sugar is in the ingredients list of almost every product in the grocery store.

If sugar is so widespread in our food system, how can it be bad? First, there is the very-powerful sugar lobby, which spends millions of dollars protecting sugar. Second, there is the misguided research by Ancel Keys from the 1960s in blaming fat for heart disease, which led food companies to reduce fats while increasing sugar content. Third, sugar has become so widely accepted in our culture that most of our holidays are sugar holidays – filled with candies, chocolates, cakes, pies, and more.

The health consequences of excess sugar consumption (and excess means more than 6 teaspoons or no more than 24 grams per day) are being seen all around us. One 12-ounce can of Coca-Cola, for comparison, has 39 grams of sugar, well over the limit – and that's just one drink out of the *whole day.*

Sugar is linked to numerous chronic and deadly diseases, including:

- Obesity
- Diabetes

- Dementia and Alzheimer's Disease
- Cancer
- Heart Disease/Cardiovascular Disease
- Stroke
- Fatty Liver Disease

Read the labels of the products you buy and stop buying products with excess sugars. Note that sugar might be listed more than once in the ingredients list (a sneaky marketing tactic) and use names that are colloquializing for sugar, usually ending in "ose" (dextrose, fructose, glucose, lactose, maltose, sucrose).

Finally, please note that natural sugar consumed in real fruits and vegetables is fine *to a degree* because the fiber therein counterbalances the sugar absorption.

> **HEALING HINT**
>
> Organic, grassfed butter from the U.S. is hard to find (please do not fall for the marketing term "European style butter"), but there are several wonderful brands from countries where pastured cows are the norm: Kerrygold (from a co-op of 14,000 family farmers in Ireland), West Gold (from New Zealand), Anchor (from New Zealand), SMJOR (from Iceland), and President (from France).

5. What are the best/worst oils to use in cooking/baking?

Regrettably, this is not a trick question, as we have been misled several times about which fats are beneficial and which ones are dangerous. We have misunderstood fats for decades, and because of that, we have badly altered the traditional ratio of omega-3 and omega-6 fatty acids in our diets.

Historically, if we look back to our ancestors (and even just a generation ago before the industrial food movement), they traditionally ate a higher concentration of foods with omega-3 fatty acids, eating anywhere from 2-4 times as much as foods with omega-6 fatty acids.

Today, because animal fats were demonized and seed oils promoted as healthy alternatives, many people are eating a ratio of 16 to 1 of omega-6 to omega-3 – or even higher. It's a major red flag and health situation because a diet high in omega-6 but low in omega-3 increases inflammation. Similarly, a diet with a balance between omega-6 and omega-3 is anti-inflammatory.

The best fat overall? Pure extra virgin olive oil. It's great in dressings as well as for cooking (at lower temperatures only). Some health experts recommend taking a tablespoon of olive oil daily. The problem is many food marketers are cutting olive oil with cheaper seed oils to squeeze out more profits. Do your research on your brand!

The best universal oil? Pure avocado oil, which is fantastic in dressings, but also excellent for cooking (especially at higher temperatures) and baking. Avocado oil has almost no taste and is extremely versatile, but again, do be careful sourcing because some avocado oils are also being cut with canola and other toxic seed oils.

Other excellent and healthy fats: virgin coconut oil, grassfed butter/ghee.

Worst oils? All the industrially-produced "seed" oils, including canola (rapeseed), corn, soybean, cottonseed, vegetable (which is always either soybean or rapeseed), sunflower, safflower, palm, and peanut.

These oils are the most dangerous/worst because they are highly processed, going through several chemical methods (including bleaching with solvents) to increase shelf life and stability… and the vast majority are made from genetically-modified plants that get doused with the toxic herbicide, glyphosate.

(According to the U.S. Department of Agriculture, GMO seeds are used to plant more than 90 percent of all corn, cotton, and soy grown in the United States, all of which are used as ingredients in the majority of all packaged foods and restaurant foods.)

If you can find cold-pressed seed oils, these are of a much higher and safer quality. Nut oils are also generally seen as safe.

Do not even think margarine over butter. Margarine, which is often used for flavoring, baking, and cooking, is most often made from toxic industrial soybean oil and/or palm oil.

6. Is meat bad for you?

If you were to believe most media dietitians and longevity experts, all meat is bad for you… which is funny, because humans have been meat-eaters almost since time immemorial.

Meat can be a great and important source of nutrients, but it completely depends on the kind of meat – how the animal is raised and sourced.

Wild game and 100-percent pastured meats are some of the healthiest foods you can eat; these meats are rich in vitamins and minerals, healthy fats, and quality protein. These are the meats that your body craves and needs – in moderation for most people.

But the meat you buy in the typical supermarket, the meat that comes from animals raised/quartered in unsanitary, unsafe, and cruel conditions is bad for more than moral/ethical reasons. Many of these animals are fed GMO grains that contain pesticides, herbicides, and antibiotics. Many of the animals are extremely young, overfed, and given growth hormones – conditions that bring more money for the big meat companies, but are harmful to consumers. Have you seen a cattle feedlot? Have you seen how industrial/factory raised chickens are housed? Sad, gross, disgusting.

Your best bet for quality meats is to find a rancher who is doing regenerative ranching and buy directly from them. Because many of us do not live near a ranch (though many of these people do sell their products at farmers markets and sometimes directly to consumers), there are organizations that work with these types of ranchers – companies such as Grass Roots Coop, Crowd Cow, Butcher Box, and others.

AUTHOR INSIGHT

Learn more details about the benefits of pastured beef in my article, Hold the BEEF! For Your Health, Eat Only Sustainable, Pastured Beef: https://www.empoweringadvice.com/grassfed-beef

7. Why should I pay more for organic produce?

Organic produce is not perfect, but when you see how many chemicals (including fertilizers, fungicides, plant growth regulators, and pesticides) are used to grow standard, conventional fruits and vegetables, you will be more than willing to pay a bit more for the organic.

Even better, find a local farmer or a farmers market where they are growing organically. (Some farmers even go beyond the organic principles without bothering to complete all the paperwork necessary to use the "organic" label.).

And if you can't afford to buy all organic produce, at least try to avoid the worst offenders, which can be found annually in the "dirty dozen" list from the nonprofit, Environmental Working Group (EWG), which uses data from the U.S. Department of Agriculture and Food and Drug Administration. According to this year's list, the most dangerous produce to buy conventionally include strawberries, spinach, kale, grapes, peaches, apples, peppers, and green beans. (Full list: https://www.ewg.org/foodnews/dirty-dozen.php)

The EWG also publishes an annual list of the 15 fruits and vegetables tested with the lowest levels of pesticide and other chemical residues, which typically includes avocados, mushrooms, pineapples, watermelons, onions, and asparagus. (Full list here: https://www.ewg.org/foodnews/clean-fifteen.php)

Researchers completing a meta-analysis of all studies focusing on organic versus conventional foods concluded: "Significant positive outcomes were seen in longitudinal studies where increased organic intake was associated with reduced incidence of infertility, birth defects, allergic sensitization, otitis media [ear infections], pre-eclampsia, metabolic syndrome, high BMI, and non-Hodgkin lymphoma." Source: https://doi.org/10.3390/nu12010007

Finally, when you can, buy organic (or naturally raised) from your local farmers market. The prices here may also be a bit higher than conventional, but you are getting the freshest and best foods while also supporting your local farmers and ranchers – truly a wonderful win-win.

Remember: Quality food is an investment in your health, so adjust your budget to put more resources into securing the *best and healthiest* food for you and your loved ones.

AUTHOR INSIGHT

My article, *Why We Need a New Victory Garden Movement,* discusses the problems with conventionally raised foods and the why and how to develop your own gardens: https://www.empoweringadvice.com/new-victory-garden-movement

8. What's the best source for healthy fresh foods?

The best source is growing your own, but because that isn't possible or realistic for many of us, the next best source is nearby farmers and ranchers and local farmers markets. The third best is buying organic at your supermarket (assuming it sells organic foods). If fresh is not a requirement, I actually prefer organic frozen because these are picked at the peak time of ripeness and then flash frozen.

But let's get back to that first and best option. Obviously, if you live in an apartment, you can't have a garden, but perhaps you can have a few window boxes of tomatoes or peppers? Or perhaps bringing together other residents to create a community garden… or there may already be a community garden established somewhere in your neighborhood. If you live in a house, then there is no excuse not to try and grow at least some of your favorite fruits and vegetables. Depending on community regulations, you could even raise a few chickens for fresh eggs.

I am also a big believer in getting to know your farmers and ranchers – whether they are local or shipping you their goods. It's important partly so you can understand and support their efforts at raising quality, clean foods, but also so that you can get tips for how best to cook the foods they raise.

Need help in finding some local farmers and ranchers? Some of my favorite sources include:

- EatWild (https://www.eatwild.com/)
- Regenerative Farm Map/Locator (https://organicconsumers.org/regenerative-farm-map/)
- American Grassfed Association (https://www.americangrassfed.org/)
- Local Harvest (https://www.localharvest.org/organic-farms/)

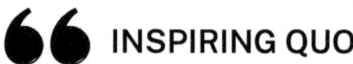

INSPIRING QUOTE

"Eat for nutrition and food value. Emphasize natural foods, avoid processed foods, and eliminate junk entirely." — Vince Gironda

9. What are ultra-processed foods, and why are they so bad?

If you buy frozen pizza or other prepared meals, or cookies and crackers, or salad dressings and other sauces… if you are buying anything with a label, it is a processed food. It becomes an ultra-processed food when the ingredients have been manipulated in such a way that they have added sugars and other questionable ingredients (dyes, preservatives, modifiers, and others) while removing the fiber (so that people eat more) and stripping away other nutrients.

About two-thirds (or higher) of the products found in traditional grocery operations are considered ultra-processed. Almost all fast foods are ultra-processed.

The four biggest issues with ultra-processed foods:

- Added sugars, to the point that we are consuming the highest amounts in human history – and food marketers hide the sugar by using multiple names for sugar in the ingredients list. Added sugar has been shown to lead to multiple health concerns, including cancer, cardiovascular disease, stroke, diabetes, dementia.
- Reduced fiber, so that the product is less filling. Daily fiber is an essential element of good health, including a healthy gut microbiome and contributing to controlling blood sugar and a healthy weight. The huge increase in colon cancer among young people is being attributed to the consumption of ultra-processed foods.
- The amount of residual pesticides, herbicides, antibiotics, and other chemicals used on the conventionally raised ingredients, including genetically-modified seeds and feed. There's concern that even in trace amounts (built

up over time) these can lead to an elevated rate of chronic diseases such as different types of cancers, diabetes, and neurodegenerative disorders.
- Questionable additives, including dyes, preservatives, seed oils, emulsifiers, and other chemicals. Many of these additives have never been tested, but have been "approved" for use. These elements can lead to increasing inflammation and reducing immune functions; additives can also cause mental health issues like anxiety, depression, attention-deficit and hyperactivity disorder, and more.

10. How healthy is fast food?

Simple answer: It is NOT healthy.

Fast food companies care about profits, thus the cheapest conventionally grown/raised foods are used in creating their offerings, and the vast majority of what is sold is ultra-processed.

All the meat, poultry, and fish come from the cheapest, industrially-raised suppliers – which means the protein you're buying is full of GMO-feed (full of pesticides, herbicides, and more), pumped with antibiotics (and perhaps growth hormones) and most likely slaughtered under stress. With the cows and chickens, most are fattened so quickly and extremely that they themselves suffer from obesity and perhaps metabolic syndrome.

The dressings and secret sauces are all ultra-processed and most contain added sugars. The breads/buns often contain sugars as well.

The fries, onion rings, and other fried items are cooked not only in toxic, industrial seed oils, but that oil is reused, reheated, reused, reheated – making the toxic oil even further degraded and disgusting. (The foods are also often coated/injected with various chemical and "natural" additives to appeal to people's tastebuds.)

The regular sodas should be called *diabetes water* (per Calley Means) for the amount of sugar in each serving – and the diet sodas are just as bad, with questionable artificial sweeteners that are linked to cancer and other health issues.

In just one meal – with a burger, fries, and a soda (or milkshake) – a person consumes 75+ grams of added refined sugar, the equivalent of 18 teaspoons… THREE times the recommended daily consumption of sugar (at about no more than 24 grams of sugar daily).

Even if you purchase a salad, which should be minimally processed, you still are eating conventionally-raised produce, which is often covered in chemicals (from pesticides, fertilizers, and herbicides like Roundup), as well as a salad dressing with added refined sugars and toxic seed oils.

FOOD FACT:
Fast foods are not inherently bad or unhealthy; it totally depends on the ingredients used and how the foods are prepared. For example, fries made from organic potatoes fried in avocado oil with added salt is perfection – three ingredients. McDonald's fries have 19 ingredients, including conventionally farmed potatoes, sugar, several toxic seed oils, and numerous chemical additives.

11. What's wrong with conventionally grown fruits and vegetables?

There are multiple reasons to avoid at least some of the conventionally raised produce – mainly dealing with the lack of nutrients and potential chemical residues – but many of these foods are also produced from genetically-modified seeds.

One of the reasons people eat fruits and vegetables is for the nutrients, including the antioxidants and polyphenols, as well as vitamins and minerals absorbed from the soil. In conventional farming, the soil has been so badly depleted that some experts say there are only about 20 years of soil left for farming. With organic – but especially regenerative – farming, the soil is healthier and contains more vitamins and minerals.

Another issue is chemical exposure. In conventional farming, many types of dangerous chemicals are used as fertilizer, herbicides, and pesticides – including the continued use of glyphosate (Roundup), which has been banned/restricted in many other parts of the world. There are more than 600 types of chemical pesticides in use with conventional farming. Organic farmers are allowed to use some fertilizers and pesticides, but they must be natural (not chemical).

According to the U.S. Environmental Protection Agency (EPA), conventional/factory farms apply a half million tons of pesticides, 12 million tons of nitrogen, and 4 million tons of phosphorus fertilizer to crops in the continental United States every year. Runoff from these applications is the leading cause of river and stream pollution, the second leading cause of wetland pollution, and the third leading cause of lake pollution.

Nitrogen alone also produces significant quantities of nitrogenous gases, including ammonia, nitric oxide, and nitrous oxide. The worst part of this practice is that about 50 percent of all nitrogen that conventional farmers use is wasted, released into the environment. Nitrous oxide is a greenhouse gas with 300 times the heat-trapping capacity of carbon dioxide, contributing dramatically to pollution and climate change.

Finally, there is the issue of genetically modified seeds. Industrial/conventional farms love using these types of seeds because they increase yields (which means more profits), help with pest resistance, and make farming easier and more "efficient."

12. Should I be following the U.S. government Food Pyramid or MyPlate?

Only if you want to keep putting on weight and using an outdated and unbalanced approach to food.

The concept has merit, but it started with flawed research that emphasized eating many daily servings of grains, breads, pastas. It was the same research that placed fat as the villain in our diet, while giving a pass to refined sugar and simple carbs – the two things we now know are driving obesity and other chronic illnesses.

Both the original Food Pyramid, which debuted in 1992, and its latest replacement, MyPlate, were designed to visually convey the elements of healthy eating to Americans of all ages. MyPlate shows four quadrants of a plate (with vegetables and grains the two biggest sections), and dairy off to the side. Bizarrely, MyPlate adds, the "hope is that the plate will nudge Americans away from meals dominated by meat and starch and towards meals made up mostly of plant-based foods."

Here's the problem. MyPlate was developed with guidance from the Center for Nutrition Policy and Promotion of the *U.S. Department of Agriculture* – not a team of expert nutritionists, but people influenced by the powerful arms of the Big Agriculture and Big Food lobbies.

Let's be clear. The government is supposed to be providing us with the best health and nutrition advice possible, but it is influenced by industry lobbyists and focused too strongly on carbs, and there is no evidence to support the idea that plant-based foods are better than pasture-raised meats on regenerative farms.

Harvard University's Healthy Eating Plate (https://nutritionsource.hsph.harvard.edu/healthy-eating-plate/) is a slightly better representation, but, again, *every person HAS to design their best plate.*

For example, "Dr. Randall's Healthy Plate," customized for my body and health, includes a larger slice of healthy regenerative meats, farm-fresh eggs, and wild-caught fish; a huge dish of nuts and seeds; a big container of healthy oils (including grassfed butter, olive oil, and avocado oil); a small mix of organic veggies; a tiny side dish of organic seasonal fruit; and a few crumbs of healthy grains. Off to the side are a large number of natural spices, including black pepper, quality salt, garlic, onion, rosemary, oregano, turmeric, cinnamon, and cayenne pepper. My glass is filled with water or my electrolyte mix.

FOOD FACT:
When buying fruits and vegetables, follow this simple rule to avoid consuming excess chemical restudies: if eating the entire item, buy organic. If it has a protective shell or peel (think avocado, banana, citrus), you can buy conventionally grown.

> **HEALING HINT**
>
> In *Why Calories Don't Count*, Dr. Giles Yeo, an obesity researcher at Cambridge University, demonstrates that the conventional model of counting calories is wrong, as all calories are not created equal. He theorizes that once people understand that calories don't count, they can begin to make different decisions about what is best for them. He states: "Calorie counting is wrong."

13. Shouldn't I be counting calories if I am trying to lose or watch weight?

Counting calories is one of the biggest wastes of time known, as is weighing your food to get the exact number of calories for each meal.

It's difficult to explain without a lot of science, but please know that all calories are NOT equal, especially in how our bodies use them. How the body utilizes the nutrients from 500 calories of broccoli is quite different than 500 calories from 2 glazed donuts; it's not the calories at all, but the *nutrient values* of the foods we eat.

The other problem with counting calories is the restrictive nature of the process – which leaves people feeling deprived, and that feeling *crushes* all dieting.

It is MUCH more important and valuable to be examining ingredient labels to avoid toxic ingredients, such as sugar, seed oils, and artificial flavors, coloring, emulsifiers, and preservatives.

Many of these ingredients are in the sugary drinks and prepared and packaged foods we buy and the fast foods we consume. Simply reducing these unhealthy products from your diet and eating more real meats, fruits, and vegetables will not only increase your health, but you will also see a reduction in your weight.

Stop counting calories and start counting grams of added sugar. In an ideal world, your refined sugar consumption should be close to zero, though even knocking it down to the government's recommended 30 grams a day would be a massive improvement.

14. What's the best way to ensure I am buying and eating healthy products?

Some of you may revolt at this answer, but the best way to ensure you are buying and eating healthy products is to purchase whole or minimally processed foods and prepare meals with them from scratch.

A generation or two ago, almost all the meals were prepared from raw ingredients, from scratch.

Today, most of our meals come from a combination of processed and ultra-processed foods, prepared meals and frozen pizzas, canned soups and sauces, fast foods, and restaurant meals (including takeout).

There are literally millions of recipes in books and online; just know you may need to alter some of the recipes to remove certain ingredients and replace with better alternatives (such as replacing seed oils with healthy oils).

Everyone can cook; it's simply a matter of following the directions from recipes. And once you get comfortable cooking from scratch, the real fun is altering recipes and trying new variations.

If you must buy prepared foods, please strive to buy organic (better, but not perfect) and follow these simple rules when examining the labels:

- Avoid foods with excessive amounts of sugar (often hidden in the ingredients list using multiple names)
- Avoid foods with unknown additives and flavorings with names you can't pronounce
- Avoid foods with more than five ingredients

66 INSPIRING QUOTE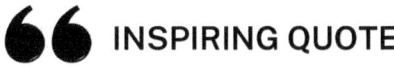

"Real food doesn't have ingredients, real food is ingredients." — Jamie Oliver

15. Is it okay to eat snacks, especially if I eat smaller meals?

Ideally, no, but it also depends on the snacks. I still remember a good friend telling me that she was a "grazer," just snacking little things all day long – and then she complained about gaining weight – though she never saw snacking (especially snacking with ultra-processed foods) as the problem.

The U.S. is a nation of snackers. We have a snacking addiction, and it's part of our current health crisis.

Back in the 1970s, almost half of adults reported not snacking between meals; today, that number is less than 10 percent.

There are two main issues related to snacking.

First, is the what. What are the snacks? Are we talking about a bowl of farm-fresh strawberries, a handful of macadamia nuts, or some grass-fed beef jerky… or, are we talking about a latte, a bag of corn chips, a package of candy, or a peanut butter and jelly sandwich? Healthy snacks may be okay for some people, the unhealthy snacks *never*.

Second, is the gut. Digestion is one of those automatic functions that begins as soon as we smell something delicious and start salivating. The issue is that digestion takes a lot of work, and if we're snacking all day long, our gut never gets a rest. One of the reasons intermittent fasting has become trendy is because we now know the importance of resting our digestive system.

Again, it comes down to your body and health. If you are a grazer of healthy foods – and it is working for you – then keep doing it. If you are a grazer and gaining weight, feeling sluggish, and dealing with brain fog – then stop grazing!

> **INSPIRING QUOTE**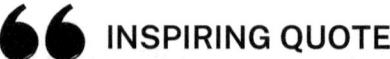
> "Sorry, there's no magic bullet. You gotta eat healthy and live healthy to be healthy and look healthy. End of story." — Morgan Spurlock

16. Can I skip breakfast? Isn't it called the most important meal of the day?

Who has not heard of breakfast being touted as "the most important meal of the day"?

Ever wonder if it's true? Most of us have heard it repeatedly and from multiple sources, right?

Big surprise: It's a marketing gimmick, like many food-related issues. It dates back to 1944, when General Foods, then the producer of Grape Nuts, wanted to sell more cereal. The advertisements stated that "nutrition experts say breakfast is the most important meal of the day."

Cereal is an $11-billion business in the U.S. According to the latest information, in 2020, more than 283 million Americans – 85 percent of the population – consumed breakfast cereals. Many of those cereals contain massive amounts of sugar; according to Scott Bruce and Bill Crawford, the authors of *Cerealizing America,* the cereal industry uses approximately *816 million pounds* of sugar each year.

Furthermore, the sugar content is much higher in children's cereals, making them more of a dessert than a meal. Amazingly, on average, children's cereals contain **40 percent more sugar** than those geared toward adults.

Besides the added sugar, most cereals are conventionally produced, using the cheapest grains (typically wheat or corn) and other questionable ingredients… grains laced with pesticides and herbicides, the fiber removed, and "fortified" with synthetic vitamins and minerals.

But it's not just cereal; we love our breakfasts. According to market research firm

The NPD Group, in 2020, people in the United States ate approximately 102 billion breakfast meals and 50 billion morning snacks.

What should you do? Find what works for you, but don't feel obligated to eat breakfast. If you do enjoy breakfast, make it a healthy one – eggs and fruit, vegetable omelet, grass-fed steak, minimally-processed organic oatmeal, or keto (no sugar) homemade muffin.

17. I don't have time to read labels when I shop. Why should I bother?

Please MAKE the time to read the labels; if you value your health, you *need* to start reading the ingredients list on all products you buy – in the store and at the restaurant.

Once you read the ingredients on that first package of crackers, cookies, salad dressing, or frozen pizza, you will never go back to not reading labels.

The three scariest ingredients in most of our processed foods, which is just about everything in your grocery store and most fast foods, include:

- **Added sugars**. The food industry has more than 70 names for sugar. Can you believe it? The reason is to help disguise just how much added sugar is in the product. All refined sugars are simple carbs and the fructose found in sugar is harmful to our bodies, and has led to the obesity and diabetes crises, as well as contributing to the mental health issues we are facing today.

- **Seed oils**. Vegetable oil? No such thing; it's typically made with soybean oil. Canola is rapeseed. All these oils are industrially produced with powerful solvents and bleaching agents. They also contribute to an imbalance in our ratio of Omega-3 to Omega-6 fatty acids. Furthermore, the raw materials (soy, corn, cottonseed) are often genetically-modified seeds and sprayed multiple times with conventional pesticides and herbicides.

- **Additives**. Food companies add all sorts of chemical substances (many untested) to the foods you buy, including dyes, spices, preservatives, emulsifiers, and other "natural" chemical flavorings. If you see items in the ingredients list you don't recognize or can't pronounce, consider not purchasing it.

Many experts suggest a five ingredient limit. Do not purchase any "foods" that need a laundry list of additives. Nature is simplicity – and all foods you eat should follow that rule.

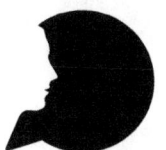

AUTHOR INSIGHT

If you're looking for more information on reading food labels, please read more in my article, Keys to Truly Understanding Food Labels: https://www.empoweringadvice.com/understanding-food-labels

18. I can't afford organic foods, what can I do? And why is healthy food so expensive?

First, no matter what you decide, you have to commit to placing a *higher value* on the food you eat. We used to spend a much higher percentage of our household income on food, but somewhere along the line, we devalued food and made other things more important – a new car, bigger house, designer clothing, expensive jewelry, lavish vacations.

Second, quality foods – whether organic or bought at a farmers market – are going to cost more than conventionally, industrially produced foods for several reasons. First, these farmers are raising the crops and animals the right way: taking care of the land, and not using antibiotics or other harsh chemicals or compounds. Also, conventional farmers can sell at a cheaper price because of their size and the fact that conventionally-raised is the mainstream – where most dollars flow. Finally, some large-scale crops are subsidized by the U.S. government.

Third, while most organic foods cost more than conventional foods, the price difference is often not that dramatically different – but the perception out there is that organic foods are widely cost-prohibitive – and that is just not the case. In fact, cooking meals from scratch with organic ingredients is often cheaper than buying prepared/packaged or fast foods (especially when you shop sales and use coupons).

Finally, organic foods may cost a bit more and you'll have to allocate more money to your food budget, but in return, you'll receive:

- Foods free of synthetic pesticides and herbicides, such as Roundup (glyphosate);
- Crops grown from heirloom and non-genetically modified seeds;
- Meats from humanely raised animals (not cruel, dirty feedlots);
- Meats from animals that aren't prematurely fattened with growth-promoting hormones and antibiotics;
- Foods that exclude many of the chemicals known as "obesogens," which trigger the body to store fat, adding to weight gain and obesity;
- Goodwill for the Earth, knowing that organic farming is widely considered to be far more sustainable than conventional farming.

19. I live in an area with limited access to quality foods, what can I do?

Food insecurity is a very sad and real situation in more parts of this country than you may be aware. Many families suffer from hidden (to us) hunger. We can make a stand by supporting community and nonprofit initiatives to end food insecurity.

This situation is the most heartbreaking to me and I greatly empathize with the plight many people and families face.

In the United States, we have both food deserts and food swamps. Food deserts are locations with limited or no grocery stores, where people have to rely on convenience stores for their groceries. Food swamps are locations with many choices of unhealthy and mostly fast and junk foods, where people are lured by the convenience, and with no other healthy choices.

Typically, the two locations that most often see one of these scenarios are Native American reservations and poor urban and rural neighborhoods.

There is no question these situations are health emergencies – and we should be doing much more to help the families barely surviving these dangerous food conditions.

Happily, several nonprofits are functioning in different parts of the country and operating on different models – with the goal of offering quality foods to people in these affected areas. My favorite is the *Food Dignity Movement*, which pays local small farmers for their goods (rather than seeking donations), and then gets the food into the hands of families in need.

Because the vast majority of the major food retailers operate on a profits-over-people mentality and refuse to operate stores in "less desirable neighborhoods," new ideas and support must come from the community and nonprofits. Food Dignity interests me because it serves two deserving populations – the small, local farmers, often struggling to make ends meet, and the families in need get access to fresh and healthy foods.

> 66 **INSPIRING QUOTE**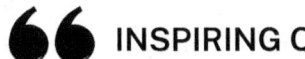
>
> "One of the forgotten links in all these food systems, connections between agriculture, nutrition, and health, is that you need knowledge. You need to do some research, and then you need to innovate ... If we can put trillions and trillions of dollars into good research on safeguarding the economy, we should also be putting in quite a bit of funding for health and food systems."
> — Ruben Echeverria

FOOD FACT:
Research shows that about 99 percent of beef in major retail supermarkets is from conventionally raised grain-fed cattle that spend about 120-200 days in feedlots, also known as concentrated animal feeding operations (CAFOs). Stuck in crowded pens, the cattle are fed a diet exclusively of grains (which is not their natural feed), and treated with hormones and antibiotics to fatten them quickly.

20. Why do some people say our food system is broken?

An entire book could be written just on this question. Our food system is indeed broken… in fact, *ruined*.

We either need an entirely new system or we have a lot of work to do to fix the current system.

We aren't eating real food anymore; the vast majority of us have unknowingly been converted to ultra-processed food junkies, with a fast food and sugar habit, eating large quantities of these imposter foods.

Starting back in the 1970s, there was a mistaken push to remove beneficial animal fats from the American diet; saturated fats were demonized, while sugars and simple carbohydrates were ignored, even considered healthy.

The vast majority of the foods in the middle of the grocery store are these ultra-processed products, which have been nutritionally (and chemically) altered to remove "bad" fats and fiber, replacing those with added refined sugars, dangerous seed oils, and a host of chemical additives.

The sugar in these products is addictive, while the lack of fiber gets us to eat more and more. The seed oils also have inflammatory effects and have completely knocked out our natural balance of omega fatty acids, important dietary fats. Because of how much processed foods we eat, we consume an abnormally high amount of Omega-6 fatty acids, which are inflammatory, and a very low amount of Omega-3 fatty acids, which are crucial for health.

The system is broken, because even if you are wise enough to skip all the ultra-processed foods in the middle of the store, the meats and produce are not much healthier – because the bulk of the meats and produce grocery stores sell come from massive, "industrial" farms and feedlots that raise their animals and crops conventionally – meaning that they often use pesticides, herbicides, and other dangerous chemicals in raising the crops and animal feeds and use antibiotics, growth hormones, and cheap, contaminated feed in raising the animals. Have you seen pictures of a feedlot?

The meats you buy from Walmart or Safeway or Winn-Dixie or Kroger or H-E-B or Costco are metabolically unhealthy; *you are eating meat from sick animals.*

The food system is broken because the entire burden of finding high-quality, sustainably-raised vegetables and meats is on the consumer.

Food marketers have *no interest i*n fixing a system that brings them massive profits, because most of the foods for sale at grocery stores and fast food restaurants are made from the cheapest ingredients.

21. As long as I exercise regularly, I can eat whatever I feel like, right?

Wrong. That would be like an addict saying as long as they are healthy and take breaks from the addiction, the drugs they are taking are perfectly fine.

Yes, food can be an addiction, especially ultra-processed grocery and fast foods. These foods have been chemically altered to enhance flavor, add sugar, and remove fiber, making them irresistible and hard to stop eating (because the fiber is what helps us feel full, satiated).

Now, even if you are eating healthy, real foods, you should not eat whatever and whenever you want. The digestive system needs time to rest/heal; it does this between meals (unless you are snacking) and at night, while you're sleeping.

But if you have a sugar/sweet tooth, then no amount of exercising will help balance the damage you are doing to your liver and gut microbiome, which are essential to health, not to mention the damage to your teeth and the effect on your mouth microbiome.

Both food and exercise/movement matter to your health and healing, as well as longevity – but it makes no sense to play one off the other. Of course, the higher the intensity of your workouts, you'll want to match your nutrition levels.

If you care about your physical and mental health, your goal should be eating high-quality foods that provide quality fuel for your body and brain, while also committing to daily movement, including both aerobic and resistance exercising.

Exercise is an essential part of a healthy lifestyle, but it has to be matched with consistently high-quality foods.

22. Should I go gluten-free or grain-free?

It depends. The debate over gluten and whether we should consume it is almost as big as the other big food controversy – whether we should consume dairy. It's also interesting to note that the rise in gluten sensitivity started about the same time our food system changed to the industrial model.

Gluten is a natural protein found in many grains; it's the element in grains that gives dough that "stickiness" and chewy factor in the baked product.

Should you consume gluten? If you can eat breads, pasta, cereals, crackers, etc., without having stomach discomfort, then there's no reason to avoid it – except for the high carb content. Gluten intolerance is small, but seems to be growing rapidly. "Gluten-free" has also become a key marketing term to lure people who are fearful of gluten; for example, potato products being labeled gluten-free (because they don't contain gluten) to attract buyers.

Some experts believe that the stomach/intestinal issues some people experience with grains comes not from the gluten, but from the vast amounts of herbicide (specifically glyphosate) used in raising the crops. The other issue is that the vast amount of wheat grown in the U.S. is not the traditional wheat our grandparents consumed, but a dwarf and semi-dwarf variety that produces a better yielding crop, but not a *quality* crop; once again, a decision made solely on profits, not crop/food quality.

Grains are not our enemy – especially whole grains – but they need to be organically-grown… and ideally, fermented.

One interesting piece of anecdotal evidence: Gluten intolerance is much lower in Europe, where most of the wheat grown is a traditional (and softer) variety; many countries in Europe have also banned some of the most dangerous pesticides and herbicides, which are still legal and used in growing U.S. grains.

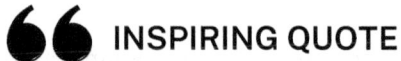 **INSPIRING QUOTE**

"Your diet is a bank account. Good food choices are good investments."
— Bethenny Frankel

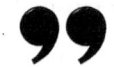

23. Should I go dairy-free?

Next to gluten, the other food with the largest amount of debates and discussions by health experts is dairy. Dairy has an interesting history – remember the Milk Mustache ad campaigns?

There's evidence that humans have been drinking cow's milk for thousands and thousands of years, with studies tracing consumption back to the Middle Neolithic period, about 6,000 years ago.

Animal milk has been a staple in homes for a long time, but that also doesn't mean animal milk is good for everyone.

Like gluten, whether you should be consuming any dairy products depends on how your body reacts to it – but it's not about the fat in dairy, which is a healthy fat; it is about the sugars and the lactose. A good proportion of the population has some level of intolerance, which can cause bloating, nausea, diarrhea, gas, abdominal pain, and vomiting.

That said, if you want some of the nutrient benefits of dairy, you might look into ultrafiltered milk, which removes much of the lactose, making it lower carb than regular milk. Ultra-filtered milk has a similar taste and often better nutrition profile than regular milk, making it a great option to explore.

As for how much dairy, the USDA (United States Department of Agriculture) recommends THREE servings of milk per day, which once again seems excessive and unbalanced.

The vast majority of the dairy in the U.S. is from cows raised conventionally on high amounts of grains (containing glyphosate and other dangerous chemicals); there is also a small amount of goat and sheep milk products (mostly cheeses or yogurts). Thus, if you choose to consume dairy products, it's best to choose milk from pastured animals from local dairies or farmers markets – or from branded products produced with grassfed dairy cows.

24. What's the one thing I should eliminate from my diet today?

Sugar. Without question, sugar is the biggest disrupter to our health – both mentally and physically.

Sugar is making us fat, sick, and depressed – and it is addictive!

Just like the tobacco industry, the sugar industry discovered decades ago that sugar has multiple health issues, and they covered up the research and paid for other researchers (including famously from Harvard University) to publish false research studies that showed sugar was fine.

Also, as with cigarettes, many experts and health officials are now suggesting that warning labels be placed on sugary, processed foods and drinks.

Let's count the ways sugar is bad:

1. Sugar is now clearly linked with multiple deadly conditions, including heart disease, stroke, and cancer. With the amount of sugar being consumed in the Western diet, it is now more deadly than cigarette smoking.
2. Excess sugar consumption is also linked to our obesity and insulin resistance problems… diabetes and dementia.

3. Our bodies have no way to process refined sugars, so it ends up in the liver, leading to multiple issues, including nonalcoholic fatty liver disease, now the most common type of liver disease.

4. Refined sugars disrupt our gut microbiome, the trillions of gut bacteria and other organisms that help with every system in our bodies, feeding bad bacteria and yeast. Excess sugar is one of the causes of something called Leaky Gut, which is when the intestinal wall weakens, leading to the possibility of toxins entering the bloodstream.

5. Refined sugars negatively impact our mitochondria, which are the energy sources found in ALL of our cells. Mitochondria are responsible for generating each cell's supply of adenosine triphosphate (ATP), a molecule that the body uses for energy. Refined sugars cause mitochondrial dysfunction, triggering cell death and provoking oxidative stress, resulting in possible muscle weakness, neurological problems, and organ dysfunction.

6. Sugar is an addictive drug, hitting the same reward center in the brain as cocaine, making it hard for many people to quit sugar. Sadly, because sugar is so pervasive in the culture, it is now being labeled as the real gateway drug leading to the use of much harder drugs, such as cocaine and heroin.

25. Should I be concerned with the lack of fiber I have in my diet?

If you are eating the conventional, standard Western diet of prepared, packaged, and fast foods, then the answer is a big YES.

Fiber is essential.

Traditionally, the nutrition profession has discussed macronutrients essential to consume as fats, protein, and carbohydrates. But with the removal of fiber from so many of the commonly eaten foods, many of us are now suggesting we need to raise the visibility of fiber, adding it as a macronutrient.

This may sound odd, but fiber is desperately needed to feed the beneficial bacteria in our gut microbiome. We are hosts to trillions of bacteria in our intestines, and their health and happiness is directly related to our health and happiness. These bacteria take the fiber and ferment it, providing beneficial and nourishing elements for our bodies and brains.

Funny aside, I remember my mom adding wheat germ to all her baked goods when I was a teenager; it became a family joke that anything she could sneak wheat germ into, she would. Guess what? She was ahead of her time! Wheat germ is a beneficial fiber, what we call a prebiotic, a food source for our gut microorganisms and which helps increase the diversity of those microorganisms.

There is a growing concern that the spike being seen in colon cancer, especially among younger adults in their 30s and 40s, is mainly due to the massive shift in our processed foods to eliminate the fiber.

Furthermore, including enough fiber in your diet lowers your risk of heart disease, stroke, high blood pressure, obesity, colorectal cancer, and gastrointestinal conditions (such as diverticulitis, constipation, and hemorrhoids).

Sadly, many people are grossly fiber-deficient.

What are some of the best sources of fiber? Seeds and nuts, whole vegetables and fruits. Some of my favorites are macadamia nuts, pumpkin seeds, chia seeds, avocados, strawberries, mushrooms, carrots, broccoli, sweet potatoes, and apples.

AUTHOR INSIGHT

For more information about fiber, please read my article, For Good Health, Please Consume Fiber! https://www.empoweringadvice.com/for-good-health-consume-fiber

26. Can my diet *really* help prevent diabetes, heart disease, cancer, and other chronic health conditions?

Yes. Unquestionably, the most important thing you can do for your health is to improve your diet.

In the U.S., we have a sickcare system, not a healthcare system. All the money goes to solving and managing symptoms from illnesses and accidents. There is no money in preventive care, thus people have to go outside the current system to learn preventive measures.

Changing from a diet high in sugary drinks, sugary snacks, and unhealthy (ultra-processed) foods to one with meals made from real ingredients, few snacks (and make them savory), and unsweetened beverages will have a profound effect on your health.

The current Western diet of ultra-processed and fast foods contains multiple health issues caused by the cheap and dangerous ingredients in these foods, including added refined sugars, industrial seed oils, and unknown/unresearched chemical additives that are known to alter fat storage and cause weight gain.

These foods have also been stripped of their natural fiber, which is yet another health danger because our digestive system needs fiber.

Your diet plays a major role in physical health; it also plays an important role in mental health. Choosing the right foods – the foods that nourish your body and mind – is critical to health.

Finally, when buying real ingredients for your cooking and baking, please try to buy from local sources (such as farmers markets) or organic because most conventionally raised produce are contaminated with the pesticides, herbicides, and other chemicals used to maximize crop efficiency and growth (without regard for what these toxins do to your health). And with purchasing your meats, again, ideally from local sources, and always grassfed, pasture-raised; for fish, always source from wild-caught; and with eggs, strive for local farm-fresh or organic at your store.

> **HEALING HINT**
>
> A larger percentage of the population is chronically dehydrated; we all need to be drinking more water and other healthy fluids. Besides negatively affecting our health, dehydration often masks itself as hunger, causing us to eat when we are simply thirsty. The next time you're feeling hungry, try drinking a full glass of water and waiting for 20 minutes; you may find you were thirsty, not hungry.

27. What role does hydration play in my health?

Hydration – proper hydration – is truly vital to health. Water serves as a key building block in all of our bodies' cells.

The recommendation is to consume at least eight 8-ounce glasses of water per day (the 8×8 rule) or drink about three-quarters of your weight in ounces per day (a 175 lb. person would consume about 14-16 8 oz. glasses), but keep in mind other sources you consume, such as soups and foods that contain a lot of water, as well as how physically active you are and the climate and temperature.

Most people do not drink enough liquids each day, and those that come close are often drinking too much sugar waters (including sodas, energy drinks, sports drinks).

Hydration/water is especially important for these functions:

- Brain health. Studies show just a slight drop in our hydration can cause impairment in many brain functions.
- Weight loss. Liquids can be very filling, so it always makes sense to drink more when attempting to lose weight. Furthermore, some studies show that increasing water intake can increase metabolism; thus, water has the potential to increase satiety and boost metabolic rate, leading to weight loss.
- Headaches and migraines. There's some evidence that dehydration may trigger some headaches and migraines.

- Bowel movements. Hydration appears to help keep constipation at least partially at bay. Increasing hydration may help decrease constipation.
- Limiting kidney stones. These very painful mineral crystals that form (and get stuck) in the urinary system may be kept under better control by keeping a high level of hydration, especially with those who have had previous bouts with kidney stones.

For most people, water is the best source for keeping hydrated. If exercising, consider adding a safe and healthy (no-sugar) electrolyte mix. (My favorite is Ultima Replenisher.) Coffee and tea, as well as coconut water, are also good sources.

28. I don't have time to cook meals from scratch. What can I do?

Snarky answer: Make the time if you truly care about your health and the health of your loved ones.

But time pressures are real, and when working long hours and/or with long commutes, it can feel like there is no time to prep a healthy dinner. There's also the energy it takes to cook a dinner, which might be hard after a long work day.

Just remember that healthy does not mean you have to make five-course meals. You can make healthy meals that do not require hours of prep work and cooking.

Here are some of my suggestions for those who want to cook meals from scratch but have limited time:

- Use days off to make big meals, guaranteeing leftovers for a future meal. For example, I cook a turkey on Sunday for dinner, then I can do several things with the leftovers – turkey soup, turkey and gravy revisited, turkey salad, turkey chili, turkey casserole, etc.
- Use a crockpot or similar device first thing in the morning to create meals that cook all day. I love how tender and juicy tougher cuts of meat become after cooking all day. Crockpot meals are also usually big enough to get two meals.
- Especially in cooler months, make big batches of hearty soup. Not only are they nutritionally-dense, but often you can get several meals from one prep.
- Use simple recipes that take no more than 30 minutes to prep and cook during some of the work days. I love to cook, but am not a sophisticated chef in the least. Some of my go-to recipes include: almond baked trout, grilled (or pan-fried in olive oil) burgers, chicken soup, eggs (with multiple variations of fried, scrambled, omelet, quiche), baked meatballs, baked chicken strips/tenders, chef salad.

- Use one of the many hundreds of recipe websites/blogs to find new and exciting meals. There are even general recipe sites as well as recipes for every type of eating/diet.

Find some of my favorite fun and easy recipes in Chapter 10.

FOOD FACT:
About 9 out of 10 Americans cook at home from scratch at least once a week, but only a quarter of Americans cook from scratch more than five times a week, according to research from Kitchen Infinity. That's not a whole lot of home cooking!

29. I am afraid of fasting, is intermittent fasting a good option for me?

Intermittent fasting is trendy these days – and many people are trying it for the many health benefits, including improving blood sugar regulation, sharpening cognitive functioning, helping heart function, inducing cell repair, reducing inflammation and oxidative stress, and increasing fat burn.

Some research suggests it even potentially increases longevity.

There's nothing new about fasting, except we have better tools for understanding how fasting works and why it provides many benefits.

Almost all our ancestors fasted – not because they were trying to be trendy – but because they were hunters and gathers with little options for food storage. If the hunting or fishing was bad, there were no meals until the next successful capture of animals or fish.

Intermittent fasting is quite different than traditional fasting methods. With intermittent fasting, people cycle between periods of eating and periods of fasting. Some do this method every day, others do it once a week, while still others, once a month. The key is finding what works for you.

The goal of intermittent fasting is to give the digestive system a long rest. The easiest method is to stop eating after 8 pm, skipping breakfast the next day, and breaking the fast at lunch (or at dinner, if doing a longer fast); doing it this way, about half your fast is while sleeping. Most experts agree that an ideal length is 12 hours, but the better benefits kick in at 14-16 hours.

When fasting, remember to increase your hydration, ideally with electrolytes. The biggest mistake people make is not drinking enough during a fast.

Consider consulting with your health provider about fasting, because even short periods of calorie restriction can result in complications for people with certain health conditions.

30. What are some simple ways I can improve my nutrition today?

The food system is so broken that health-focused consumers unfortunately have to take extra time researching and sourcing nutrient-dense foods.

All these efforts can seem overwhelming, so here are a few suggestions for getting started:

- Find and shop at a local farmers market. (Many now take debit/credit and SNAP, so cash is not always necessary.)
- Switch out one or more sugary drinks with water. (If plain water gets boring, infuse yours with natural herbs or bubbles or buy one of the many unsweetened flavored water brands; my current favorite is Topo Chico Sabores.)
- Buy more organic products, and when possible, use frozen organic produce because these items are harvested and frozen at peak ripeness. (Many fruits and vegetables are harvested prior to ripeness to allow time for thousands of miles of transport.)
- Switch out sugary snacks with savory, such as salted nuts and seeds. Not only will this reduce your sugar intake, but nuts and seeds are excellent forms of fiber, of which many people are deficient.
- Switch out industrial vegetable (seed) oils, which are contaminated with solvents and pesticides from genetically modified seeds, and high in the wrong kind of fat (Omega-6), with beneficial and healthy oils, such as pure olive oil, avocado oil, coconut oil, or grassfed butter.
- Reduce your purchases of packaged and prepared foods and fast foods. These products have been overly processed (ultra-processed) to the point where they should have warning labels. These products have added sugars, use bad oils in place of good fats, include conventionally raised ingredients (often filled with pesticides, herbicides, antibiotics, and other chemicals), sprinkled with questionable chemical additives, while stripping most of the beneficial fiber.
- Add one additional meal made entirely from scratch – using healthy, real ingredients.

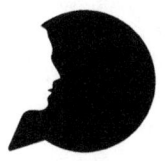

AUTHOR INSIGHT

For more information on fasting, please see my article, Are You Utilizing the Power of Intermittent Fasting? https://www.empoweringadvice.com/utilizing-the-power-of-intermittent-fasting

31. What's up with all this talk about the gut microbiome?

For so many years, doctors and scientists focused on the heart and the brain as the two key centers of our bodies, but over the last decade or so, the focus has been on the gut and how it influences so many functions in the body.

At first, the gut was being called our "second brain," but today, many are saying the gut is our primary brain, with the actual brain more like a computer processor that takes inputs from the gut and our senses.

Even though the "grandfather" of modern medicine, Hippocrates, stated more than 2,000 years ago that all disease starts in the gut, the role of the gut has been mostly ignored and replaced by a conventional medical model that focuses almost exclusively on symptom management, not curing/healing.

All of us have trillions of friends living in and on our bodies mostly in the form of bacteria, but also viruses, yeasts, and other micro-organisms. We know there is a gut microbiome, a skin microbiome, a mouth microbiome – and some are suggesting there is also a brain microbiome.

In the gut (specifically the intestines), these bacteria – including the balance of beneficial and harmful bacteria – play a role in many aspects of our health, especially metabolic health.

The gut microbiome plays a role in digestion, metabolism, immunity, emotions, and mental health. We now know that most of our immune cells are in the gut and that most of the serotonin (a chemical messenger that affects mood, cognition, sleep) produced in our bodies is NOT in our brain, but from the gut microbes!

The gut microbiome has also gotten more attention recently because of the change in our diets over the last 50 years. Researchers have found that the Standard American Diet of fast and ultra-processed foods, along with a host of other factors (including the overuse of antibiotics and other medications), have led to a less diverse gut microbiome and a *starving* gut microbiome.

Read more about the gut microbiome in Chapter 2.

32. Fermented foods seem really trendy, especially with longevity, are they healthy?

Before there was any kind of refrigeration, many people used fermentation to help preserve foods for future consumption. But since the time of electric refrigeration – about a century ago – many people have moved away from fermenting their foods.

Some cultures have continued using fermented foods, and that combined with the interest in the gut microbiome have led to renewed interest in the role of fermented foods on health.

Research now shows that a diet rich in fermented foods enhances the diversity of gut microbes, enhancing the strength of the gut microbiome.

The greater the health and diversity of the gut microbes, the stronger our immune system, the better our mental health, and the more efficient our digestion and metabolism.

Many fermented foods are considered natural probiotics because they help improve and restore the gut microbiota.

Some common fermented foods you may be aware of include yogurt, sauerkraut, miso, kefir, kimchi, and kombucha. Pickles and sourdough bread are also fermented.

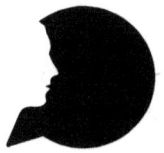

AUTHOR INSIGHT

One of my favorite fermented foods that I use in a variety of recipes is apple cider vinegar, which you can buy in bottles at many stores – or try making it yourself. If you buy it from the store, please make sure it is organic and contains "the mother," which is the beneficial bacteria. I used to buy Bragg's exclusively, but since the family sold out, I have switched to Fairchild's Organic Apple Cider Vinegar, which many consider to have the best quality and taste.

33. What is metabolic health and its relation to metabolic syndrome?

Metabolic health deals with how well your metabolism is working; metabolism is your internal process that converts food into energy the body can use.

Metabolic health has become the canary in the coal mine; that is, when we have multiple markers showing poor metabolic health, it is a precursor to a host of chronic physical illnesses, including diabetes, non-alcoholic fatty liver disease, cancers, dementia and Alzheimer's disease (now being called type 3 diabetes), cardiovascular diseases like heart attack and stroke, and chronic kidney disease. It has also been shown to be connected to a host of mental illnesses, including depression, anxiety, neurocognitive disorders, and attention deficiency.

Metabolic health has gained traction for the same reason as the gut microbiome and mitochondria; for a healthy metabolism, people need a healthy and diverse gut microbiome. Furthermore, the quality of metabolism has a direct impact on the mitochondria, which are the energy powerhouse of our cells. (Both the gut microbiome and mitochondria are discussed in more detail in Chapter 2.)

> **HEALING HINT**
>
> Making changes, especially in diet and lifestyle, can be overwhelming... which is another reason some diets fail. Instead, try making small, incremental changes over the course of several months. For example, just eliminating sugar may be a several-month project because it is insidiously prevalent in our food system.

The best way to support metabolic health is to avoid foods that spike blood glucose, such as foods high in sugar and simple carbohydrates, which include almost all ultra-processed and fast foods. (Other ways to support metabolic health include getting good quality sleep, reducing stress levels, and avoiding environmental toxins, especially those chemicals that disrupt the endocrine/hormone system.)

The way doctors and scientists measure metabolic health is by using these five elements:

1. **Blood pressure**. Having hypertension, or high blood pressure (130/85 or higher), which about half the U.S. population has, is a negative sign of metabolic health. You can easily measure this for yourself.

2. **Waistline**. We used to talk about body mass index (BMI), but researchers have found that simply measuring the waist is better. Having a waistline above 40 inches for men and 35 inches for women is a negative sign of metabolic health; this is another easy thing to measure for yourself.

3. **Fasting glucose**. Indicates how much sugar is in the blood after a period of no eating and only water consumption. Levels under 100 mg/dL are considered healthy; 100-125 mg/dL is considered prediabetic, and anything over 100 is considered a negative sign of metabolic health. This can easily be measured with a blood test – either with an at-home kit or a blood draw by a health professional.

4. **Triglycerides**. These are fats found in your blood, and play an important role in healthy body functions – until they become too concentrated. Triglycerides have been misunderstood for many years, in terms of the role they do or do not play in cardiovascular disease, but in terms of metabolic health, anything about 150 mg/dL is considered unhealthy. This level can only be measured with a blood panel done by a health professional.

5. **HDL Cholesterol**. Please note that much of what we once thought we knew about cholesterol has now evolved, including the role that dietary cholesterol plays in levels of cholesterol in the body. Also note that this is HDL, the supposedly "good" cholesterol. In the case with HDL, low numbers are the concern, so a result of 40 mg/dL or less is considered unhealthy.

34. What are the best foods/diet for women in perimenopause and menopause?

Finally, this topic – a challenging time in the lives of all women – is being supported with more research and in-depth examination. I have my wonderful partner and experts like Dr. Mary Claire Haver (@drmaryclaire on Instagram) to thank for really opening my eyes to how little we really know about the massive impact of menopause on women's health.

There are actually three stages to menopause, starting with perimenopause, which usually starts when women are in their forties. It typically begins eight to 10 years before menopause, when the ovaries gradually produce lower amounts of estrogen, a key hormone.

Menopause is when the woman hasn't had her menstrual cycle for 12 consecutive months, and typically occurs in the early 50s. It's when the ovaries are no longer releasing eggs and no longer producing estrogen.

The final stage of menopause is postmenopause, which lasts for the remainder of the woman's life. In the first few years after menopause, women can still experience menopausal symptoms (such as hot flashes, emotional instability, brain fog, decreased libido, sleep disturbances, and fatigue/reduced energy).

Women in postmenopause are known to be at risk for multiple health conditions, including: osteoporosis (weakening bone density), heart disease, urinary incontinence, urinary tract infections (UTIs), and vaginal infections.

The most important nonfood action women should research is hormone replacement therapy. Years ago, through more faulty research that received too much attention, doctors recommended against any kind of hormone replacement. Today, finally, with better research, hormone replacement is gaining traction – and the earlier in the stages of menopause, the better. Talk with your OB/GYN or naturopath.

In terms of diet, the big breakthrough that has been discovered thus far is the importance of two things:

- **Healthy protein.** Menopausal women need much more protein in their diets to help build muscles because one of the biggest dangers of menopause is the loss of muscle mass. Strong muscles are essential for good health. Healthy proteins (whether plant-based or animal-based) need to be added to *every* meal.

- **Non-inflammatory foods.** Menopausal women need to avoid foods that add to gut issues and chronic inflammation, which is at the core of the Healing Revolution Diet. This means cooking more from scratch with real foods and avoiding the long list of inflammatory foods, which include all sugars, seed oils, ultra-processed packaged and frozen foods, and most restaurant foods. As an aside, healthy, pasture-raised beef is not inflammatory, but conventionally-raised meats are. You'll also want to focus on having a much better balance of more omega-3 fatty acids over omega-6 fatty acids; most people on a Western diet have a massive imbalance, consuming many more omega-6 than omega-3.

Healing the gut is essential to reducing inflammation in the body.

> **HEALING HINT**
>
> If you suffer severe bloating, gas, diarrhea when eating certain foods, you might want to look into an elimination diet called FODMAP, which stands for fermentable oligosaccharides, disaccharides, monosaccharides, and polyols – carbs found in foods that some people find hard to digest. It is a short-term plan to clear your gut for a few weeks, and then slowly adding back foods to see how your gut reacts. Learn more: https://www.healthline.com/nutrition/fodmaps-101

35. Besides food, what other things can I be doing to improve my health?

Heal yourself. Healing past trauma wounds and reconnecting with yourself (perhaps for the first time in many years) is the very best thing you can do along with changing your diet. If you are on medications, many can be reduced or eliminated with both a healing and health journey.

Healing trauma is at the core of my first two books – and it is essential if you want to live your optimal life. Many people either disregard/ignore past trauma or simply don't recognize that they have experienced trauma. And just FYI, we have ALL experienced some form of trauma in our lives.

When we are dealing with unhealed trauma wounds, we are overly reactive (triggered), emotionally dysregulated, and suffer with mental and physical conditions.

Bad foods and other unhealthy habits become comforts and escapes for us, thus a healthy diet will never be effective until you find healing.

A healing journey can easily be done alongside a health journey, and while it might make things a bit bumpier in the short-term, it will be life-changing in the long-term.

The great thing about healing is that you do not need to find a healer; we have our own internal healer, but it's been deactivated.

Using the tools described in my first two books and summarized in Chapter 7, you can move forward with integrating your entire past with your present, healing yourself and finding yourself.

Besides healing your past trauma, other important changes include daily movement (throughout the day), resistance training, reducing/eliminating stress, and regular, good sleep. Quitting cigarettes and reducing alcohol consumption are also vital to health and longevity.

99 INSPIRING QUOTE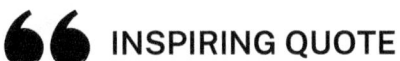

"Awareness is the first step in healing."
— Dean Ornish

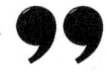

CHAPTER NINE
Health, Nutrition, and Diet Do's and Don'ts

 INSPIRING QUOTE

"Quite literally, your gut is the epicenter of your mental and physical health. If you want better immunity, efficient digestion, improved clarity and balance, focus on rebuilding your gut health." — Kriss Carr

DO start making food a priority and as an investment in your health and healing. Food is the top factor affecting our health and longevity, yet many have food as a "low-budget" item. Change that.

DON'T follow any more fad diets; these are only temporary aids to weight loss, not for supporting health.

DO build or join a supportive community, which is vital for all aspects of health and healing. A healing and health journey can be turbulent at times, and the support of your loved ones is essential to your success.

DON'T eat at fast food restaurants, which make mostly ultra-processed foods from the cheapest ingredients. One example: McDonald's fries have 19 ingredients, including added sugar.

DO start cooking more from scratch, which is the best tools for creating the healthiest foods. These meals do not need to be elaborate or time-consuming; many meals can be made from scratch in under 30 minutes and others can be slow-cooked all day in a crockpot. *See Chapter 10 for some of my favorite recipes.*

DON'T buy most conventionally-raised meats, vegetables, and fruits, because these products are inundated with chemicals, from pesticides to hormones and antibiotics. With the animals, they are often fed an unnatural diet to fatten up while being stressed from tight quarters in feedlots.

DO consume more healthy fiber, which has been found lacking in more than 90 percent of all diets because ultra-processed foods remove the fiber. Fiber is such an important nutrient, especially for our gut microbiome.

DON'T count calories. It's a waste of time, even though every single food label, by law, has to list the calories. There is a big difference between calories in the food (listed on the label) and the actual usable calories – the concept of caloric availability.

DO find for yourself the best balance of animal- and plant-based foods for optimal health – and only obtain those foods from quality sources.

DON'T fall into the cholesterol trap, another misguided theory. So much disinformation is still being published, but the key is dietary cholesterol is **not** a concern for most people.

DO embrace healthy fats of all kinds, including plant-based and animal fats; we are deficient in fat because of so many "low-fat" ultra-processed foods. Healthy saturated fats do **not** cause plaque or heart disease, as was thought incorrectly for decades.

DON'T consume any simple carbohydrates, eliminating all sugars and white flours. Simple carbs have no real use for most people, converting quickly into sugar in your body. If you choose to eat carbs, focus on more complex carbs, which take longer to digest.

DO decide for yourself whether gluten and dairy are good or bad for your health. The debate over these two items is still being hotly debated. If you can eat foods with gluten and lactose and experience no side effects (such as bloating and stomach pain), then do so, but make sure you are buying organic.

DON'T drink sodas, juices, and other sugary beverages, which some have labeled "diabetes water," and are major drivers of the obesity and chronic health crisis.

DO stay hydrated, including drinking a glass of water about 30 minutes before every meal. Drink lots of water; you can add natural flavors or even bubbles to make it more appealing. Consider using a safe (no-sugar) electrolyte brand to up the value of your hydration. Remember too that people often eat when the body is actually dehydrated – not hungry. The standard recommendation that you should modify based on your circumstances: males should consume 15.5 cups of water daily; females about 11.5 cups daily, dependent on weight, weather, exertion.

DON'T snack all day long; it's a dieting urban legend; snacking all day spikes blood sugar, possibly leading to insulin resistance. In fact, most nutrition experts suggest eliminating most daily snacking as well as shortening the time window of when we eat, from the typical 12 hours to something like 8 hours (or even shorter, especially when using intermittent fasting).

DO add more vegetables to your meals; they add both nutrients and fiber to your diet, but remember to find the vegetables that your body most needs and that do not produce side effects (such as from lectins and oxalates).

DON'T eat dessert for every meal, which is currently happening because so much of the food available to us in grocery stores and restaurants has high amounts of added sugars.

DO start reading ingredient labels and changing buying habits, which should be a key step in your health journey; awareness of the many sugars and chemical additives will change your buying habits.

DON'T simply replace sugar with questionable sugar substitutes, especially those in the convenient yellow, pink, and blue packets. Try stevia or allulose, or simply try eliminating all sweeteners.

DO cook big batches of foods for second, third meals – as a convenient way during the work week to have some simple meals that just need reheating for a healthy dinner.

DON'T use any "vegetable" seed oils, which are produced in a toxic chemical process using both bleach and solvents and contain high levels of Omega-6 fats and linoleic acid, which are considered inflammatory.

DO use healthy oils and fats in place of those "vegetable" seed oils. Healthy oils and fats include grassfed butter, olive oil, avocado oil, coconut oil, and ghee.

DON'T eat ultra-processed foods, which are the bulk of the items in your typical grocery store – including almost all the food items on the shelves and in the frozen section. These are the foods that are the leading cause of our health and obesity crisis.

DO shop at famers markets and food co-ops, which usually not only have the freshest and healthiest foods, but by doing so, you also support the local farmers in your community.

DON'T consume refined sugars. Stop all (or as much as possible) sugar use, which has been a known toxin and additive substance for more than 60 years. Fructose (from sugar) is a poison in our bodies, especially our livers.

DO eat more nuts and seeds, which contain many beneficial nutrients as well as being a wonderful and healthy source of fiber.

DON'T fall for food marketing gimmicks, such as "all natural" or "heart-healthy" or "antibiotic-free" or "important source of vitamins and minerals." These statements have no meaning or value but are meant to trick you.

DO eat more mushrooms, avocados, and eggs – as long as your body and gut thrive on them; these three are true superfoods, packed with so many nutrients and beneficial elements for our bodies and brains.

DON'T eat too much fruit, which does have a place in most diets because of the nutrient value, but remember they have a high (natural) sugar content that makes them to be eaten in moderation for most.

DO buy organic whenever possible. Yes, you will pay more for the products, but you will be avoiding so many chemical contaminants and genetically-modified elements found in conventional foods.

DON'T ignore the advice of adding more fermented foods into your diet; eating some fermented foods aids and strengthens your gut microbiome.

DO consider growing some of your own food, whether that's a big garden in your yard or a window box in your apartment – or a plot in a community garden. Eating freshly picked foods is truly magical – providing you with the highest levels of nutrients.

DON'T always eat breakfast; consider intermittent fasting, which gives our digestive system a longer and restorative rest between eating. Skipping breakfast occasionally is the easiest way to do a short fast.

DO understand that our food system is horribly broken, focused on producing low-nutrient and highly-addictive foods produced from the cheapest conventionally-grown ingredients. Most of the hundreds of food brands are owned by a handful of conglomerates focused purely on profits and shareholder wealth.

DON'T forget to clean up the nonfood areas of your household, including removing as many chemical products as possible, starting with air fresheners, carpet cleaners, antibacterial soaps, and more.

DO develop a diet based on how your body, brain, and gut react to foods – which is the basic premise of the Healing Revolution Diet. Everyone needs to develop a customized diet based on how their bodies react to certain foods.

DON'T stop seeking health and healing knowledge because we are continuing to make breakthroughs and gain new understanding of how we can all live our best and healthiest lives.

DO consider getting bloodwork done to test for vitamin and mineral deficiencies, as well as the basic metabolic panel (BMP) and lipid panel, which examine blood glucose, cholesterol, and triglyceride markers.

DON'T allow yourself to become overwhelmed when making changes to your diet. Take one step at a time in your health journey, starting with one change and slowly making others. Remember, it is a journey and not a race.

DO heal your past trauma wounds, which may be driving some of your food addiction and other struggles. If we can both fix our food debacle AND heal from our past trauma, then the sky is the limit in terms of a long and productive and happy, love-filled, and peaceful life!

FOOD FACT:

Another label to look for – and avoid buying. Some producers are using Apeel, a plant-based protection that was developed "to help keep produce stay fresh for longer." Unfortunately, many health experts are sounding the alarm, saying that the product contains trace amounts of lead, cadmium, arsenic, palladium, and mercury – all heavy metals. Learn more: https://www.saintjohnsorganicfarm.com/articles/is-apeel-safe

PART TWO: HEALING REVOLUTION DIET TOOLS

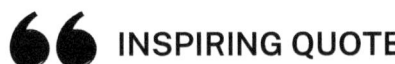 **INSPIRING QUOTE**

"It's all about nutrition. You can train, train, train all you want, but I always say you can't out-train a bad diet." — Joe Wicks

CHAPTER TEN
Healthy and Easy Recipes

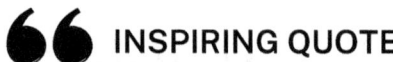 **INSPIRING QUOTE**

"The second day of a diet is always easier than the first. By the second day you're off it." — Jackie Gleason

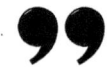

The following pages contain a number of my favorite recipes that I make regularly.

These recipes are not meant to be exhaustive, but to be a model for the types of recipes and foods you can be making for yourself and your family.

You'll notice that the vast majority of my recipes are simple and fast. No one will ever accuse me of being a gourmet, and I don't care because my focus is on health, not the perfect display and plating of meals.

Thousands and thousands of recipes exist online – and for every diet type. I encourage you to explore and keep growing your repertoire of favorite meals to cook and eat!

Finally, all I can add is make the creating, cooking, baking, and eating a family-fun experience. I learned to cook in my mom's kitchen and to this day, I love making nourishing and healthy meals for my partner.

Stop by prepared foods and explore the wonders and delights of home cooking and baking!

A final note about the tools that will aid you greatly in cooking healthy, nutritious, and delicious meals at home. I recommend these items; you do not need all of them now, but they are a convenience to cooking, so consider some of these an investment in your health as well.

KEY KITCHEN TOOLS

- Good set of knives and a knife sharpener
- Set of quality cutting boards
- Large skillet and saucepan with ceramic coating; ditch the no-scratch chemical surfaces
- Cookie sheet/baking pan set
- Unbleached parchment paper (stop using aluminum foil)
- Strong blender; Vitamix is perhaps the best brand in this category
- Set of 3-4 ceramic (or metal) mixing bowls of various sizes
- Electric mixer and/or immersion blender
- Wooden spoons, spatulas, flippers
- Crockpot or instant pot
- Vegetable steamer
- Glass measuring cups
- Metal measuring spoons
- Indoor electric grill

Healthy, Hearty, and Easy Chili

What follows is an easy recipe for a healthy, hearty, and keto-friendly chili. Makes 4 servings, but consider doubling the recipe so that you have leftovers! Prep time is about 15 minutes; cooking time is 15-25 minutes.

INGREDIENTS

- Avocado or olive oil (for sauteing)
- 1-2 pounds grassfed ground beef (can mix and match; 1 lb. ground beef; 1 lb. stew meat) – or organic ground turkey
- 1 red or orange bell pepper (cut up)
- 4-5 cloves garlic (crushed)
- 1 cup chopped mushrooms (sliced/chopped)
- 1 medium onion (chopped)
- 4 green onions (sliced thinly)
- 2 14-oz. cans of organic diced tomatoes
- 1 can (small) organic tomato paste
- 3/4 cup organic beef bone broth
- Slurp of red wine (about a quarter cup)
- 1 teaspoon red pepper flakes
- 1 teaspoon chili powder
- 1 teaspoon cumin powder
- 1/2 teaspoon turmeric powder
- Salt and pepper to taste

DIRECTIONS

1. Sauté onions, garlic, pepper, and mushrooms in oil in a large pot.
2. Remove those and place them aside, leaving the oil in the pot.
3. Sprinkle salt, and pepper on the beef.
4. Brown beef.
5. Add the remaining ingredients to the pot, stirring thoroughly.
6. Depending on your schedule, cook on medium heat for 15-20 minutes.
7. When ready, serve the chili in a bowl, and add optional ingredients.

OPTIONAL INGREDIENTS

- 1 avocado
- 1/2 cup of shredded organic cheese
- Organic sour cream at serving

Hearty and Healthy Crockpot Beef Stoup

What follows is an easy crockpot recipe for a healthy and hearty beef soup... or stoup. Makes 4 servings, but consider doubling the recipe so that you have leftovers! Prep time is about 15 minutes; crockpot time is about 9 hours on low or 5 hours on high.

INGREDIENTS

- 2-3 pounds of grassfed beef (cubes or cut up into bite-sized pieces)
- 4 tablespoons of organic/grassfed butter
- 1 large onion
- 4 cloves of garlic, minced
- 2 cups carrots (sliced, diced)
- 1/2 cup of finely diced celery stalks
- 8 ounces of mushrooms, sliced/diced
- 2-3 cups of organic beef broth
- 1-2 cups of green beans or broccoli (chopped)
- 1-2 bay leaves
- 1/2 cup dry red wine (optional)
- 1 14-oz can of organic diced tomatoes
- Salt and pepper to taste

DIRECTIONS

1. Sauté onions, garlic, and mushrooms in butter in a large skillet.
2. Remove those and place them aside, leaving the butter in skillet.
3. Sprinkle salt, and pepper on the beef pieces.
4. Brown beef on both sides in the same skillet, adding additional butter or olive oil. About 10 minutes or so.
5. Repeat for all beef pieces.
6. Throw beef and the remaining ingredients into your crockpot.
7. Depending on your schedule, cook on high (5 hours) or low (9 hours).
8. When ready, serve the beef stoup in a bowl.

Delightful and Spicy Thai Red Chicken Curry

What follows is a very easy recipe for making the best all-natural spicy red curry chicken – with no added sugars, preservatives, or other ingredients. It takes about 10-15 minutes to prepare and another 15-20 minutes to cook.

INGREDIENTS

- Avocado or coconut oil
- 1 large organic onion, diced
- 2 organic red, yellow, orange peppers, diced
- 1" of ginger root, cut into tiny pieces (do not peel ginger root)
- 3-4 garlic cloves, crushed (depending on how much you like garlic)
- 2 cans of organic coconut cream
- 1 block of organic creamed coconut, 7-ounce box (for added creaminess)
- 2 organic chicken breasts, cut into small pieces
- 2-3 tablespoons of red curry paste
- 1/2 teaspoon cayenne pepper
- 1/4 teaspoon chili powder (optional)
- 2 teaspoons basil
- 4 teaspoons liquid coconut aminos
- 1 lime
- 1 can of bamboo shoots
- 1 8-ounce package of mushrooms, sliced
- 1 teaspoon Himalayan sea salt to taste
- Optional: Water chestnuts for more crunch

DIRECTIONS

1. Using a large pot, cook chicken in avocado (or coconut) oil; set aside.
2. Sauté mushrooms; set aside.
3. Sauté peppers for 2-4 minutes; set aside.
4. Sauté onion, garlic, ginger, cayenne pepper.
5. Add in the remaining ingredients: coconut cream, chili powder, coconut aminos, basil, bamboo shoots.
6. Return mushrooms, peppers, and chicken to mix.
7. Simmer lightly for 6-10 minutes.
8. Let cool for about 5 minutes; squeeze lime, stir, and serve.
9. (Add additional cayenne pepper or curry paste to raise the «heat.»)

Consider other options; *for Thanksgiving, we used organic turkey breast rather than chicken breast. We also add an 8-ounce organic riced broccoli to enhance the curry. And in the most recent version, we also added dried Aronia berries (a super antioxidant).*

Creamy, Nutritious Super Green Soup

What follows is an easy recipe for making one of my favorite soups; you literally feel yourself absorbing the nutrients. Takes about 45 minutes to prep and cook. Makes 6 servings.

INGREDIENTS

- 1 large organic broccoli head, cut up (or 2 cups of frozen organic broccoli florets)
- 2 cups of organic spinach
- 2 cups of organic mushrooms
- 10 tablespoons of organic butter
- 2-3 cloves of garlic, minced
- 10 green onions
- 3 cups of organic chicken broth
- 1/2 cup coconut milk (or organic heavy cream)
- 2 cups of shredded organic "Mexican blend" cheese

DIRECTIONS

1. Sauté broccoli, spinach, onions, garlic, and mushrooms in butter in a large skillet on medium heat for about 15 minutes.
2. Remove those and place them into a high-powered blender.
3. Add to blender, coconut milk, and chicken broth.
4. Blend well until smooth consistency.
5. Pour the blended mix into a large saucepan, add the cheese, and cook on low heat for about 10 minutes, until serving temperature.

Optional: For added protein punch or simply for flavor, consider adding about 1-2 cups of shredded organic cooked chicken to the soup, either before or after blending.

Spicy and Smooth Coconut Carrot Soup

Here's an easy recipe to make a delicious and nutritious soup. Makes 10 servings.

INGREDIENTS

- 2 tablespoons of coconut oil (or avocado oil)
- 2 pounds of organic carrots
- 1 large organic onion
- 4 celery stalks
- 6 cups of organic chicken broth
- 1 can of unsweetened coconut milk
- 1/4 cup ginger
- 2 teaspoons of ground turmeric
- 2 teaspoons of ground cumin
- 2 teaspoons of ground coriander
- Salt and pepper to taste
- 2 tablespoons of lime juice

DIRECTIONS

1. Put carrots, celery, and ginger into food processor to make a pulp.
2. Sauté the mix with the coconut oil in a large skillet on medium heat for about 15 minutes.
3. Add the spices to the mix, stirring constantly. Cook for about 2 minutes.
4. Mix in the broth and coconut milk and raise heat to bring the soup to a boil.
5. Reduce heat and let the soup simmer for about 20 minutes.
6. Just before serving, stir in the lime juice.
7. Serve.

***Optional**: Top the soup with some toasted organic pumpkin seeds.*

Healthy Beef Heart and Mushroom

Our ancestors ate the entire wild animals they killed, something called nose-to-tail cooking, honoring the entire animal by utilizing all the parts in food preparation. Today, while nutritionists profess the value of eating organ meats, many shy away. This recipe will change your mind. It takes about 15 minutes of prep time, and another 45 minutes for cooking. Makes 4 servings.

INGREDIENTS

- 1 grassfed, pastured beef heart, cubed
- 1 1/2 cups of edible, organic mushrooms
- 1 yellow or white onion
- 1 1/2 cups of chopped tomatoes
- 1/2 cup of dry red wine
- 1 cup of organic beef bone broth
- 4 carrots, peeled and diced
- 3 cloves organic garlic
- 1 sprig of rosemary
- 3 sprigs of thyme
- 2 bay leaves
- 3 cups water
- Avocado oil

DIRECTIONS

1. Add a tablespoon or oil to a large saucepan or Dutch oven on medium heat.
2. Sauté onions and mushrooms; set aside.
3. Add a bit more oil and sauté heart.
4. Return mushrooms and onions.
5. Mix in all the remaining ingredients: carrots, tomatoes, wine, bone broth, spices, water.
6. Reduce heat to low; cover and simmer 30-45 minutes.
7. Remove bay leaves.
8. Plate in deep plates or shallow bowls.

OPTIONAL

- Consider adding a diced organic potato to make the meal even heartier.
- Cook in a slow-cooker rather than a pot.
- Use butter to help thicken the "stoup."
- If the rubbery texture of heart bothers you, cream the heart, mushrooms, and onion in a high-powered blender.

Interested in learning more about organ meats? Read: Definitive Functional Medicine Guide To Organ Meats (https://drwillcole.com/food/the-complete-functional-medicine-guide-to-organ-meats)

Chunky Turkey Soup Provencal

This tasty soup has a French-herb influence that will make it stand out from other soups. Takes about 40 minutes to prep and cook. Makes 4 servings.

INGREDIENTS

- 1 pound of ground organic turkey breast
- Olive or avocado oil
- 1/2 teaspoon of dried herbs de Provence, crushed
- 1 clove of garlic
- 1 small organic white/yellow onion
- 1 can (14 oz) of organic diced tomatoes
- 4 cups of fresh spinach
- 1 cup of organic chicken or turkey broth
- Salt and pepper to taste

DIRECTIONS

1. Mince/cut garlic.
2. Dice onion.
3. Heat skillet to medium with oil, add onion and garlic; sauté for 5 minutes.
4. Add ground turkey (putting more oil in skillet as needed) and brown thoroughly.
5. Mix in spices, tomatoes and broth; raise heat; stir well.
6. Add in spinach, reduce heat, and let simmer for five minutes.

Optional: *The traditional recipe is normally made with cannellini beans, but kidney beans also work well for those who want beans in their soup.*

Smooth Sweet Potato and Mushroom Soup

This amazing soup combines two powerful foods, sweet potatoes and edible mushrooms, both loaded with nutrients. Plus, multiple options make this soup a great staple for dinners. Takes about 45 minutes to prep and cook. Makes 6 servings.

INGREDIENTS

- 4 tablespoons grassfed butter or avocado oil
- 1 medium organic white/yellow onion
- 3 garlic cloves, minced
- 1 cup of celery
- 1-2 sweet potatoes (enough to make 2 cups)
- 2 cups of organic mushrooms
- 6 cups of broth (chicken or vegetable best)
- 1/2 teaspoon cinnamon
- 1/4 teaspoon nutmeg
- 1-2 teaspoons Himalayan (or other healthy) salt
- 1 teaspoon freshly ground black pepper
- 1/2 cup unsweetened coconut milk

DIRECTIONS

1. Chop onions, celery, mushrooms, and potatoes. Mince garlic.
2. Heat butter/oil on medium-high heat in a large pot and add onion, celery, and garlic; cook for about 5 minutes, stirring frequently.
3. Add mushrooms, as well as salt and pepper; cook for about two minutes.
4. Pour broth over the entire mix; add cinnamon and nutmeg, stirring; turn heat to high, bring broth to boiling.
5. Add the potatoes and immediately lower to medium heat, simmering for about 12-14 minutes.
6. Throw pot ingredients into a blender or use immersion blender in pot; blend until smooth.
7. Pour soup back into the pot; add coconut milk while heating.
8. Taste soup and add any additional spices for taste.

Optional: *You can add carrots or other favorite veggies, as well as a healthy protein (such as chicken, turkey, or tofu) to make it more of a "stoup." Try additional healthy spices, such as rosemary, thyme, or turmeric.*

Prep Hint: *You can easily cut and chop the ingredients the day before or the morning before, storing the ingredients in the fridge in airtight containers until ready for cooking.*

Keifer-Infused Chicken Stoup

Here's another way to use leftover chicken breast – whether oven-cooked or grilled – adding a little fermented goodness (and tang). Fast meal! It takes about 10 minutes to complete this recipe, with 10 minutes of cooking time. Makes 2-3 servings.

INGREDIENTS

- 1 cup of diced, cooked organic chicken breast
- 1 cup of edible organic mushrooms, sliced
- 2-3 organic green onions, sliced
- 2 cups of fresh organic spinach
- 1/2 cup finely chopped/shredded organic carrots
- 1/2 stick grassfed butter or equivalent avocado oil
- 1/2 cup of organic plain Keifer
- Lime juice for taste
- Salt and pepper to taste

DIRECTIONS

1. Melt butter on medium heat and sauté green onions and mushrooms for about 8 minutes.
2. Add spinach and carrots and continue cooking for 4 minutes, until spinach is wilted.
3. Throw in the chicken and spices.
4. Add Kiefer and sprinkle with lime juice.
5. Simmer for a few minutes.
6. Serve in a bowl or deep plate.

Optional: *Some interesting ideas to change up the traditional salad:*

- Add diced broccoli florets
- Add some garlic and/or pepper flakes for added spice
- Add shredded organic cheese for taste and as a thickener

Fast and Easy Spatchcock Roast Chicken

The classic slow-roasted chicken is hard to beat, but this recipe makes delicious roasted chicken in about half the time! With this recipe, the chicken is thoroughly cooked, but with no dried out and overcooked parts. Perhaps the hardest part of making a spatchcock chicken is the little bit of butchery needed, including having a sharp boning knife or kitchen shears to do it. You can also use this same recipe for spatchcocking a turkey. Takes about 65 minutes to prep and cook. Makes 6 servings.

INGREDIENTS

- 1 whole farm-fresh or organic chicken
- 2 tablespoons olive oil
- 1 tablespoon of toasted garlic flakes or garlic salt
- 1 packet of chicken herbs, or freshly harvested rosemary, sage, and thyme
- Salt and pepper

DIRECTIONS

1. Preheat oven to 440 degrees.
2. Place the chicken onto a cutting board, breast side down. Use a boning knife or kitchen shears to cut away the spine.
3. Flip the chicken over, breast side up, and crack the breastbone to open the chicken (like laying a book down).
4. Place the flattened chicken on a cooking rack situated on top of a baking sheet.
5. Situate herbs under the chicken.
6. Massage oil onto all areas of the chicken. Top with salt, pepper, and garlic.
7. Place chicken in oven and roast for about 30-40 minutes.
8. When done, take chicken from oven and let rest on counter before carving.

Optional: Consider roasting some sweet potatoes or toasted brussels sprouts at the same time as roasting the chicken.

Delicious and Amazingly Simple Ran Burgers

So many people have complimented me on these burgers, but it's not what I do to them, but the type of meat, which is of course pasture-raised and grassfed beef. It's a simple recipe. I grill the burgers, but they could also be pan-fired or cooked in the oven.
Takes about 45 minutes to prep and cook. Makes 3 servings.

INGREDIENTS

- 1 pound of grassfed ground beef
- 1 tablespoon olive oil
- Salt and pepper
- Onion and/or garlic salts
- Optional spices and rubs, such as Everything But The Burger Seasoning

DIRECTIONS

1. Light grill or preheat oven to 400 degrees.
2. Prep the ground beef by forming it into three patties
3. Coat one side with olive oil and then sprinkling spices.
4. If using the oven, prepare a baking sheet with parchment paper and add burgers.
5. For the grill, once preheated, place the oil side of burgers on the grill.
6. After about 7 minutes, flip the burgers.
7. Continue cooking until desired state of pinkness.

Optional: Turn the burgers into cheeseburgers by adding your favorite organic cheese about 5 minutes before you plan to remove the burgers from cooking. You could also consider sautéing or grilling an organic onion and/or with mushrooms and other organic veggies to enhance the goodness!

Scrumptious and Simple Baked Chicken Breast

A simple and quick way to get a home-cooked meal on the table. This dish was my go-to for many years when I was working two jobs and had a family to feed. It's a simple recipe, taking just a few minutes of prep time. Takes about 40 minutes to prep and cook. Makes 4 servings.

INGREDIENTS

- 4 locally-grown or organic chicken breasts
- 1 tablespoon olive or avocado oil
- Salt and pepper
- Optional spices and rubs, such as Spice Hunter Organic Poultry Seasoning

DIRECTIONS

1. Preheat oven to 400 degrees.
2. Line a baking dish or small cookie sheet with parchment paper.
3. Place chicken breasts in dish and coat one side with oil, salt and pepper, sprinkling spices.
4. Bake for 30 minutes or until the center of breasts reaches 160 degrees.
5. Remove chicken from oven and let rest, covered, for about 10 minutes.

Optional: *Consider these options:*

- Adding a slice of organic cheese (about 5 minutes before removing from oven), such as Havarti, provolone, or mozzarella
- Make them spicy by sprinkling chili powder, garlic powder, or other herbs/spices
- I sometimes add a cream cheese and spinach stuffing to this recipe – by slitting the breasts in the middle to create a pocket, and stuffing with the mixture. (Doing this may add a few more minutes to your baking time.)

Mediterranean Tomato Almond Mushroom Chicken Strips

This recipe is a such a treat for the mouth and the gut! Simple ingredients and short cook time make it perfect for a workday dinner. Takes about 30 minutes to prep and cook. Makes 2 servings.

INGREDIENTS

- 2 organic chicken breasts, cut into strips
- 1 medium organic red bell pepper, diced
- 8 oz organic edible mushrooms, sliced
- 2 cups of organic cherry tomatoes
- 1 cup of organic sliced almonds
- 1/2 teaspoon garlic powder
- 1/2 teaspoon oregano
- Salt and pepper to taste
- Olive oil

DIRECTIONS

1. Preheat oven broiler.
2. Spray/coat a baking dish or small cookie sheet.
3. Place cherry tomatoes, garlic, and salt in dish and place about 8 inches from broiler.
4. Flip every five minutes, cooking for about 15 minutes until some of tomatoes start to blacken.
5. At the same time, put a tablespoon of oil in a saucepan over medium heat and sauté almonds until browned.
6. Remove the almonds, add more oil to the pan, and sauté the mushrooms.
7. After the tomatoes are done, switch oven to bake at 425 degrees.
8. Place chicken strips on parchment-lined baking sheet and sprinkle with spices.
9. Bake for about 12 minutes.
10. Serve tomato mixture topped with toasted almonds and cooked chicken.

Optional: Consider these options:

- Make the strips spicy by sprinkling chili powder, garlic powder, or other herbs/spices
- Throwing in some spinach as the base for the dinner, plating first before adding tomatoes and chicken and almonds

Super Easy and Delicious Trout Amandine

This recipe is a healthier twist on the classic recipe! Simple ingredients, hearty-healthy fish, and on the table in under 20 minutes. Takes about 20 minutes to prep and cook. Makes 2 servings.

INGREDIENTS

- 2 wild-caught steelhead trout fillets
- 1/2 cup of sliced almonds
- 2 tablespoons butter
- Salt and pepper
- Organic parsley flakes

DIRECTIONS

1. Preheat oven to 350 degrees.
2. Place fillets on a small baking sheet lined with unbleached parchment paper.
3. In a small saucepan, melt butter with almonds, until lightly brown.
4. Carefully pour the almonds and butter mixture over the trout.
5. Sprinkle salt, pepper, and parsley on the trout.
6. Cook for about 10 minutes, until fillets turn pink and almonds are toasted.

Optional: *You can also use an organic fish spice mixture, such as Mama Patierno's Organic Chicken & Poultry Spice Rub.*

Magnificent Oven-Baked Macadamia-Encrusted Fish

This amazing dish can be prepared in under 30 minutes!
Takes about 30 minutes to prep and cook. Makes 4 servings.

INGREDIENTS

- 4 "white" wild-caught fish (mahi-mahi, haddock, cod, halibut, sea bass) fillets
- 1 tablespoon olive or avocado oil
- 1 cup of roasted macadamia nuts, reduced to bits in food processor
- Garlic powder/salt
- Salt and pepper to taste
- Fresh lemon or organic lemon juice

DIRECTIONS

1. Preheat oven to 425 degrees.
2. Prepare a small baking sheet with parchment paper.
3. Prepare macadamia nuts until all that's left is small crumbs.
4. Place crumbs on a small dish big enough for dipping each fillet.
5. Coat one side of a fillet with oil and push into crumbs; place crumb side up on baking sheet.
6. Repeat with remaining fillets.
7. Sprinkle with salt, pepper, garlic.
8. Place in oven for 12* minutes.
9. Switch to broiler and brown the top of the fillets lightly, no more than 2 minutes.
10. Plate fillets and squeeze lemon juice onto each fillet.

Optional: *This recipe works for other fish as well. For example, we have made this recipe with salmon. For a more tropical taste, you can reduce the amount of nuts and add unsweetened coconut flakes.*

* Bake time depends on the thickness of the fillets. A general rule of a thumb is that fish needs about six minutes of cook time (at 425°) per every half-inch of thickness... plus an extra minute or two, as needed.

Bountiful Bison Mouthwatering Meatballs

Who wants hearty and beneficial bison meatball dish in under 30 minutes!
Takes about 30 minutes to prep and cook. Makes 4 servings (of about 20+ meatballs).

INGREDIENTS

- 1 pound of ground bison (though you could also use grassfed beef or pastured turkey)
- 1/2 cup of chopped carrots
- 1 cup cut up zucchini
- 1 cup of chopped kale (stems removed)
- 1/4 cup of raw almonds
- 1/4 cup of chopped onion
- 1 garlic clove
- 1-2 teaspoons of Italian seasoning (to taste)
- Salt and pepper to taste

DIRECTIONS

1. Preheat oven to 375 degrees.
2. Prepare a baking sheet with parchment paper.
3. In a food processor or powerful blender, lightly puree carrots, kale, and almonds.
4. Add remaining ingredients, except for the meat, and blend lightly.
5. Move wet mash into a bowl and add meat, mixing well.
6. Using a small ice scoop or your hands, create small meatballs and place on baking sheet.
7. For something a little different, place some shredded cheese on top of each meatball.
8. Place in oven for 10 minutes.
9. Roll meatballs and cook for another 10 minutes.
10. Plate meatballs and drizzle with Ranch dressing or a simple tomato sauce.

Moist and Tasty Ground Turkey Mini Loaves

Speaking from personal experience, many people avoid making meatloaf because they are often extremely dry, even without overcooking. This recipe solves that problem by making several mini loaves rather than one big meatloaf. Takes about 40 minutes to prep and cook.
Makes 6 servings (of about 4 mini loaves).

INGREDIENTS

- 2 pounds of ground pastured turkey (though you could also use pastured chicken)
- 1/2 cup of chopped carrots
- 3 pastured, organic eggs
- 1 1/2 cups of finely chopped organic mushrooms
- 1 medium onion, finely chopped
- 1/4 cup of chopped onion
- 1 garlic clove, minced
- 2 tablespoons organic tomato paste
- 1 tablespoon of organic mustard
- 1-2 teaspoons of Italian seasoning (to taste)
- Salt and pepper to taste

DIRECTIONS

1. Preheat oven to 375 degrees.
2. Prepare a baking sheet with parchment paper.
3. In a large bowl, mix together all ingredients.
4. Separate mixture into four equal parts and form the loaves on baking sheet.
5. Place in oven for 30 minutes.
6. Remove from oven and serve.
7. Consider drizzling with organic sour cream, Kefir sour cream, Ranch dressing, a simple tomato sauce, or a sugar-free ketchup.

Deliciously Chessy Oven-Baked Organic Eggs

Looking for a new way to have your eggs? Tired of fried or scrambled? What follows is an easy recipe for making delicious and fun baked eggs. It takes about 30 minutes to complete this recipe, with 10 minutes of prep time, up to 15-20 minutes for baking.

And please do NOT be afraid of eggs, especially organic or farm-fresh eggs, which are a superfood! Eggs contain all sorts of nutrients, including: Vitamin A, folate, pantothenic acid, vitamin B12, riboflavin (vitamin B2), phosphorus, selenium, vitamin D, vitamin E, vitamin B6, calcium, and zinc. Pastured eggs are also high in Omega-3 fatty acids. Finally, do not be concerned about any issues regarding the past lies about the dangers of cholesterol from eggs.

INGREDIENTS

- 6 organic eggs
- Organic avocado or olive oil cooking spray
- Salt & pepper, other spices
- Onion flakes
- Cheese (slab or shredded)
- Garlic Gold Seal Salt Nuggets

DIRECTIONS

1. Preheat oven to 350 degrees.
2. Prepare 1 muffin pan.
3. Spray pan with avocado or olive oil spray.
4. Drop the eggs into the muffin pan. (Optional: you can scramble the eggs if you prefer)
5. Add spices, cheese
6. Place in oven for 15-20 minutes (partly dependent on how you want your egg yolk)
7. Cool for 5 minutes before serving.

Organic Crustless Keto Cheesy Quiche

What follows is an easy recipe for making delicious natural, organic, low-carb crustless keto quiche. It takes about 15 minutes of prep time, and another 35 minutes for baking. Makes 1 - 8 x 8 pan or 9-inch pie-dish Quiche.

INGREDIENTS

- 5 farm-fresh eggs
- 1 medium organic onion, diced
- 3-4 heads of organic garlic, minced
- 8 oz. of fresh or frozen organic spinach
- 1/2 cup cream, milk, or coconut milk
- Pinch of salt, pepper, or other favorite spices
- 1 cup shredded organic cheese (or slices) - Havarti, Monterey Jack, Mexican blend

OPTIONAL INGREDIENTS

- 1 cup of diced organic chicken, turkey
- 12 slices of organic, no-sugar bacon
- 1-2 summer organic or wild-game sausage (depending on size)
- 1 cup sliced/diced organic mushrooms

DIRECTIONS

1. Preheat oven to 375 degrees.
2. In a skillet, add avocado oil and cook onions, garlic, fresh spinach, mushrooms.
3. Spray cooking dish/pan with organic olive or avocado oil and add ingredients from the skillet.
4. Add bacon, sausage, or other meats to dish/pan.
5. Crack open the eggs in a large mixing bowl.
6. Using a whisk, mix together eggs, spices, and milk/cream.
7. Pour egg/milk liquid over the ingredients in pan/dish.
8. Cover the top layer of pan/dish with cheese.
9. Bake for 35 minutes, or until top is golden brown. (If it browns too quickly, put foil over the top of the pan/dish.)

Optional: *If you really desire a crust, you can use almond and coconut flour (with egg and butter) to make a crust... but try it crustless first and you may never miss having a crust.*

*Heavenly and Delicious Chicken Fricassee**

What follows is a very easy recipe for making one of my mom's favorite dishes – chicken fricassee. Makes 4 servings, but consider doubling the recipe so that you have leftovers!

INGREDIENTS

- 4 organic pasture-raised chicken breasts (or one whole chicken, cut up)
- 4 tablespoons of organic/grassfed butter
- 1 small onion
- 10 pearl onions
- 3 cloves of garlic, minced
- 2 celery stalks, chopped
- 1 cup of finely diced or julienne organic carrots
- 8 ounces of mushrooms, sliced/diced
- 2 cups of organic chicken broth
- 1/4 cup coconut milk (or organic heavy cream)
- 1/2 cup dry white wine
- 1 teaspoon of poultry seasoning
- 2 sprigs of fresh parsley
- 2 sprigs of fresh thyme
- 2 tablespoons of arrowroot (for thickening sauce)
- Salt and pepper to taste

DIRECTIONS

1. Sauté onions, garlic, and mushrooms in butter in a large skillet.
2. Remove those and place them aside, leaving the butter in skillet.
3. Sprinkle poultry seasoning, salt, and pepper on the chicken pieces.
4. Brown chicken on both sides in the same skillet, adding additional butter or olive oil. About 10 minutes or so.
5. Repeat for all chicken pieces.
6. Throw all the chicken and onion/garlic/mushroom mix into a large pot.
7. Add carrots, celery, and herbs.
8. Add wine and broth to the pot.
9. Bring the entire mix to a boil, then reduce heat to let simmer for about 25-30 minutes.
10. When ready, remove the chicken pieces and add arrowroot to thicken the sauce.
11. Taste the sauce and supplement with salt and pepper or other spices as needed.
12. Add chicken back to pot and let sit for a few minutes.
13. Plate the chicken fricassee in a bowl or lipped plate.

Optional: *Cook up some organic spinach (butter or olive oil in the skillet with the spinach, which will reduce dramatically) and use the spinach as the base for the chicken fricassee.*

*This is a modified and healthy version of my mom's favorite meal!

Decadent and Delicious Waldorf Chicken Salad

I didn't learn of the deliciousness of Waldorf Salad until late into my adult life, but better late than never, right? The easiest time to make this recipe is after you have made a roast chicken (or turkey). Fun trivia: The Waldorf salad was first created in 1893 by Oscar Tschirky, the first maître d' of New York City's Waldorf Hotel. It takes about 15 minutes of prep time, assuming the chicken has been cooked beforehand. Makes 4 servings.

INGREDIENTS

- 1 1/2 cups of cooked chicken (typically breast meat)
- 6 stalks of organic celery
- 1-2 organic gala or fuji apples (depending on size; 1 medium-sized is enough)
- 10 romaine lettuce leaves or butter lettuce
- 1/2 cup toasted walnuts
- 1/2 cup of homemade or organic, avocado or olive oil mayonnaise
- 1 tablespoon of lemon juice
- Salt and pepper to taste

DIRECTIONS

1. Cube/chop chicken into bite-sized pieces.
2. Core and cut apple into bite-sized pieces.
3. Cut celery into small pieces.
4. Cut walnuts into small pieces.
5. Rip apart or cut romaine into small pieces.
6. Toss all ingredients into a big bowl, mix, and salt and pepper to taste.

Optional: *Some interesting ideas to change up the traditional salad:*

- Add diced avocado to the salad.
- Add some organic sour cream or organic yogurt.
- For a little spice, add some crushed red pepper flakes or diced jalapeños.
- Substitute apple with a cup of raspberries or blueberries for a change and a pop of color.
- Throw in some other veggies, such as diced red onions, sliced radishes, or diced cucumber.
- Try wild-caught salmon instead of poultry for a different taste.

Spicy Chicken Keto Taco Salad

Instead of all the carbs and chemicals in tacos, this recipe uses a lettuce wrap for a wonderfully healthy and fun dish. It takes about 15 minutes of prep time, assuming the chicken has been cooked beforehand. Makes 4 servings.

INGREDIENTS

- 2 cups of cooked chicken (typically breast meat), diced
- 1 avocado, diced
- 1 red bell pepper, diced
- 1/4 cup organic salsa
- 1/2 cup organic shredded Mexican blend cheese mix
- Salt and pepper to taste
- 4 romaine lettuce leaves or butter lettuce
- Optional spices and rubs, such as Riega Organic Taco Seasoning or organic chili flakes

DIRECTIONS

1. Dice top four ingredients and throw into a large mixing bowl.
2. Add salt and pepper to taste.
3. Prepare lettuce.
4. Scoop chicken taco mix onto lettuce leaves.
5. Sprinkle with cheese.
6. Serve cold.

Optional: *Some interesting ideas to change up the traditional salad:*

- Add some organic sour cream or organic yogurt.
- For a little more spice, add some crushed red pepper flakes or diced jalapeños.
- For more nutrients, throw in some sliced black olives and/or black beans.
- Try wild-caught salmon or trout instead of poultry for a different taste.

Home-Style Smothered Meatballs Casserole

Here's a modern, healthy, and keto twist on the classic spaghetti and meatballs, but without the toxic white pasta. This one is full of grassfed ground beef, tomato, and cheesy goodness! It takes about 15 minutes of prep time, and about 45 minutes of cook time. Makes 6 servings.

MEATBALL INGREDIENTS

- 2 pounds of ground grassfed beef (or substitute with chicken or turkey)
- 1 cup of shredded mozzarella cheese
- 1 cup of shredded zucchini
- 1 egg
- 2 teaspoons of minced onion
- 3 teaspoons of minced garlic
- 2 teaspoons of basil
- Salt and pepper to taste

SAUCE INGREDIENTS

- 1 28-ounce can of organic crushed red tomatoes
- 3 cloves of garlic, finely chopped
- 1/2 small organic onion, diced
- 1/4 cup of extra virgin olive oil
- 1/2 tsp oregano
- 1/2 teaspoon rosemary
- 1 teaspoon of crushed red pepper flakes
- Salt and pepper to taste

TOPPING INGREDIENTS

- 8 oz shredded Italian cheese

DIRECTIONS

1. Preheat oven to 400 degrees.
2. Spray or coat a casserole dish with avocado or olive oil cooking spray.
3. Combine all the ingredients for the meatballs and mix thoroughly.
4. Using a tablespoon or ice cream small ice cream scoop, form about 24 meatballs and place them in the casserole dish.
5. Bake for 30 minutes, then temporarily remove from oven and drain the excess liquid from the casserole dish.
6. While meatballs are cooking, get a medium saucepan for the preparing the sauce.
7. Sauté the garlic and onion in the olive oil. Be careful not to let it burn.
8. Add the tomatoes, salt, pepper, and herbs to the saucepan. Let simmer for 5-10 minutes, allowing the sauce to thicken a little.
9. With the sauce completed, pour over cooked meatballs and add shredded cheese topping.
10. Bake for an additional 10-15 minutes or until the cheese is melted.

Tasty and Simple Roasted Brussels Sprouts

Perhaps you love them, but for me, I had too many boiled ones in my childhood to never want to eat them again. But, thanks to my brother-in-law, I tried these roasted brussels sprouts and found them wonderfully tasty. Takes about 45 minutes to prep and cook. Makes 6 servings.

INGREDIENTS

- 1 1/2 pounds brussels sprouts, ends trimmed and yellow leaves removed
- 3 tablespoons olive oil
- 1 teaspoon Himalayan (or other healthy) salt
- 1/2 teaspoon freshly ground black pepper

DIRECTIONS

1. Preheat oven to 400 degrees.
2. Place all ingredients into a large resealable plastic bag. Seal tightly, and shake to coat.
3. Pour the coated sprouts onto a baking sheet, and place on center oven rack.
4. Roast for 30 to 45 minutes, rotating sprouts every 5 to 7 minutes for even browning.
5. The sprouts are done when brown, almost black.

Organic Buttermilk Ranch Salad Dressing

What follows is a fairly simple recipe for making the best all-natural buttermilk ranch dressing – with no added sugars, preservatives, or other ingredients. It takes about 5-10 minutes to prepare (a bit longer if you make your own mayo and buttermilk) and is ready for use or can be chilled for later use. I suggest placing the dressing in several mason jars.

INGREDIENTS

Purchase organic ingredients to keep your salad dressing as clean as possible.

- 1 jar of 32 oz. healthy mayonnaise (or make your own*)
- 2 1/2 cups of organic buttermilk (or make your own**)
- 3 teaspoons of minced dried onion
- 10 tablespoons of dried parsley
- 3-4 teaspoons of minced garlic or Garlic Gold nuggets (or five small cloves of garlic, minced, with 1 tablespoon of avocado or olive oil)
- 1/2 teaspoon of crushed chili flakes and/or chili hot sauce
- 1 teaspoon of freshly ground pepper
- 1+ teaspoon Mrs. Dash "Table Blend" or similar to taste
- 1 teaspoon Himalayan (or other healthy) salt to taste
- 1 16 oz sour cream (or make your own***)

DIRECTIONS

Put all the ingredients in a bowl, starting with the mayonnaise and buttermilk, and blend together with a whisk. Ladle into vessels and refrigerate.

OPTIONS

1. Make your own mayonnaise, but you need an immersion blender and...
Mix the first five ingredients; then very slowly add the oil as you are blending until you get a rich and creamy blend.

- 3 eggs (room temperature)
- 1/2 teaspoon of mustard
- 1/2 teaspoon of sea salt (or other salt)
- 1/2 teaspoon of pepper
- 1/4 cup lemon juice
- 1-1/2 cups avocado oil (simply the best; or high-end olive oil)

2. Make your own buttermilk...
Pour lemon juice into the milk, mix, and let stand for about 10 minutes. Done.

- 1 cup of whole milk, organic when possible (or half-and-half or heavy cream)
- 1 tablespoon of lemon juice

3. Make your own Kefir sour cream...
Split heavy cream into two mason jars; add half of Kefir into each jar; mix, seal, and refrigerate after letting jars sit overnight on the counter.

- 1 16 oz. organic, grassfed heavy cream
- 6 tablespoons of plain, no-sugar, organic Kefir

Tangy and Clean Thousand Island Salad Dressing

Want a fun and tangy salad dressing – with no added sugars, preservatives, or other ingredients? Look no further! This dressing has a fascinating history that started on a cruise along The Thousand Islands, a region on the upper St. Lawrence River. It just so happens that the owner of the Waldorf (yes, of Waldorf salad fame) was on board and brought the dressing back to the hotel, where it grew in popularity.

It takes about 5-10 minutes to prepare (a bit longer if you make your own mayo and buttermilk) and is ready for use or can be chilled for later use. I suggest placing the dressing in several mason jars.

INGREDIENTS

Purchase organic when possible

- 1 jar of 32 oz. healthy mayonnaise (or make your own*)
- 1 cup of organic no-sugar ketchup, such as Primal Kitchen, Unsweetened Ketchup
- 1 16 oz. container of sour cream
- 1/2 cup of apple cider vinegar
- 1/2 cup of minced onion flakes
- 1/2 cup of minced (sweet or dill) pickles
- Garlic (minced or flaked) to taste
- Salt and pepper to taste

DIRECTIONS

Put all the ingredients in a bowl, starting with the mayonnaise and ketchup, and blend together with a whisk. Ladle into vessels and refrigerate.

OPTIONS

*Make your own mayonnaise, but you need an immersion blender and...

Mix the first five ingredients; then very slowly add the oil as you are blending until you get a rich and creamy blend.

- 3 eggs (room temperature)
- 1/2 teaspoon of mustard
- 1/2 teaspoon of sea salt (or other salt)
- 1/2 teaspoon of pepper
- 1/4 cup lemon juice
- 1-1/2 cups avocado oil (simply the best; or high-end olive oil)

Delicious and Nutritious Crispy Kale Chips

Here's how to easily make delicious kale chips! What follows is an easy recipe for making delicious and crispy kale chips. If you have never had these, they are a wonderfully healthy and salty snack! It takes about 20 minutes to complete this recipe, with 10 minutes of prep time, up to 10-12 minutes for roasting. Kale is truly one of the best foods you can eat... high in antioxidant vitamins A, K, and C, as well as a good source of minerals, including copper, potassium, iron, manganese, and phosphorus. Kale may provide significant health benefits, including cancer protection and lowered cholesterol. Kale chips make an amazingly better substitute for other salty snacks, such as chips. (And for you gardeners, kale is VERY easy to grow!)

INGREDIENTS

- 10+ stalks of kale leaves
- Organic avocado or olive oil cooking spray
- 1-2 teaspoons of Garlic Gold Seal Salt Nuggets* (or use plain sea salt, or cayenne pepper or taco seasoning, or chili powder)

DIRECTIONS

1. Preheat oven to 350 degrees.
2. Prepare 1 or 2 cookie sheets.
3. Spray cookie sheet(s) with avocado or olive oil spray.
4. Remove kale leaves from stems, tearing into bite-size pieces. (Do not wash kale; if needed, do so earlier if necessary and let dry.)
5. Spray the kale with olive oil spray.
6. Sprinkle Garlic Gold* sea salt nuggets – or your topping of choice – on the kale pieces.
7. Place in oven for 8-10 minutes.
8. After 8 minutes, check kale for crispiness; rearrange and put back in oven for another 5 minutes – or until kale pieces are all dry, crisp.

Buttery Garlic-Infused Buttered Spinach

Spinach is such a versatile and nutritious vegetable (except for folks sensitive to oxalates) that can be used in many recipes. Here is a simple standalone scrumptious spinach side dish. Find your fresh spinach at the farmers market, grow your own, or buy organic. It takes about 7-8 minutes to complete this recipe, with 1 minute of prep time, up to 6-7 minutes for cooking. Note: It will look like a LOT of spinach when you first start this recipe, but spinach cooks down dramatically. Makes 6 servings.

INGREDIENTS

- 2 large bunches of fresh, organic spinach
- 4 cloves organic garlic, thinly sliced
- 2 tablespoons melted grassfed butter
- 1 teaspoon lemon juice
- Salt and pepper to taste

DIRECTIONS

1. Heat butter in a large sauté pan or skillet. Sauté garlic until aromatic.
2. Add spinach; drizzle with lemon juice and stir to combine well.
3. Continue to sauté until the spinach starts to wilt. Do NOT overcook.
4. Season with salt and pepper.
5. Transfer to a serving plate.
6. Garnish the spinach with lemon wedges and serve immediately.

Nutritious and Mouthwatering Baked Sweet Potato Fries

Sweet potatoes are one of my favorite sources of fiber and nutrients, such as beta carotene, vitamin C, manganese, and potassium. And these baked sweet potato fries make an excellent side dish – and a bit more playful than just a baked potato. It takes about 10 minutes of prep time, up to 20 minutes for baking. Makes 2 servings

INGREDIENTS

- 1 large organic sweet potato
- 2-3 tablespoons of arrowroot powder (such as Jiva Organics Organic Arrowroot Powder)
- Avocado oil
- Salt to taste

DIRECTIONS

1. Preheat oven to 415 degrees.
2. Prepare a baking sheet by coating lightly with avocado oil.
3. Carefully slice baked potato twice – to cut into small fry "wedges." Hint: These potatoes are tough to cut, so we use a small meat/cheese slicer to slice the whole potato, then cutting each slice into "wedges."
4. Place potato wedges in bowl. Add a light coat of avocado oil and mix thoroughly.
5. Add arrowroot powder and mix again.
6. Season with salt.
7. Cook 10 minutes on bottom rack.
8. Move sheet to upper rack and cook about 9 minutes, checking not to burn the fries.
9. Transfer to a serving plate.

Optional: *You can also throw in some of your favorite spices, perhaps some chili pepper, for more spicy fries.*

Devilishly Delicious Keto Deviled Eggs

Now that we know eggs (at least farm-fresh, organic eggs) are wonderful for our health – one of the handful of superfoods – this recipe provides a dish that you can eat for breakfast, as a mid-day snack, or as a quick appetizer when friends visit. It takes about 40 minutes to complete this recipe, with 15 minutes of cooking time, 15 minutes for cooling, and about 10 minutes to assemble.
Save time by boiling the eggs the day before.

INGREDIENTS

- 8 hardboiled* eggs, cooled
- 1/3 cup of organic avocado or olive oil mayonnaise (or make your own; see the Ranch Dressing recipe) – or substitute organic plain Greek yogurt for more of a tang or mashed avocado
- 1 teaspoon of spicy or yellow mustard
- 1/4 teaspoon of garlic powder
- 1/4 teaspoon of onion salt
- Salt and pepper to taste
- Paprika (for accent)

DIRECTIONS

1. Cut peeled eggs in half lengthwise.
2. Remove yolks and place in a medium bowl.
3. Add mayonnaise, mustard, and all spices except the paprika, and mash and mix until creamy.
4. Scoop yolk mixture and place into hallowed out eggs.
5. Sprinkle with paprika.

OPTIONS

Personalize your deviled eggs with other possible ingredients, such as adding:

- Organic bacon crumbles
- Curry powder
- Wasabi paste
- Basil pesto
- Splash of lemon juice

* If you struggle with making hardboiled eggs, try this variation: Pour an inch of water into a pot and insert a steamer basket and bring water to a boil. Lower the temperature to medium-low and place the eggs in the steamer basket, cover, and steam for about 15 minutes. If you don't have a steamer basket, try steaming the eggs in a half-inch of water. The trick is that the steam penetrates the shell a bit making the eggs easier to peel. If still hard to peel, try cracking shells and leaving the eggs in a bowl of water for about 15 minutes before attempting to peel again.

Tasty Treat Keto Almond Flour Waffles/Pancakes

Love waffles and pancakes? Try this delicious, all-natural, no-dairy, organic, keto-friendly waffle/pancake recipe using almond flour, coconut milk, avocado oil, flaxseed. It takes about 10 minutes of prep time, and another 4 minutes for cooking. Makes 8 waffle squares or 12 pancakes.

INGREDIENTS

- 5 eggs
- 1/4 cup avocado oil
- 1/2 cup unsweetened coconut milk
- 1/4 cup water
- 1 teaspoon vanilla extract
- 1/2 cup ground flax seeds or hemp seeds
- 1-1/4 cups almond flour

DIRECTIONS

1. Preheat waffle or pancake grill.
2. Crack open the eggs in a large mixing bowl.
3. Using a whisk, mix together all the liquid ingredients.
4. Add flaxseed/hemp.
5. Add almond flour, adding slightly more or less, based on batter consistency.
6. Ladle onto griddle for 3-5 minutes, depending on temperature; flip pancakes halfway through.

OPTIONS

Enhance the flavor with one or both of these options:

- 1 teaspoon almond extract
- 1-2 tablespoons cinnamon

For fluffier waffles, separate the yolks from the egg whites, placing the egg whites in a separate bowl. Once the main batter is ready, whip up the whites into a stiff froth and fold into the batter.

RECOMMENDED ENHANCEMENTS

- Pure, salted butter (such as Finlandia, Kerrygold, Plugra brands)
- RxSugar Organic Flavored Syrup Maple or Lakanto Maple-Flavored Syrup
- Fresh or frozen berries
- Homemade whipped cream (heavy cream, vanilla, and powdered erythritol)

Delicious No-Sugar Classic Cheesecake

What follows is a very easy recipe for making delicious no-sugar, keto cheesecake or cheesecake muffins. It takes about 15 minutes of prep time, and another 40 minutes for baking the cake or 18-20 minutes for baking muffins. This recipe is for a basic, no-sugar keto vanilla cheesecake or cheesecake muffins with no crust/base.

INGREDIENTS

- 3 (8-ounce) packages of organic cream cheese, softened to room temperature
- 1 cup of erythritol granular (you could also use Allulose, Stevia, or other non-sugar sweetener)
- 2 large eggs
- 1 teaspoon pure vanilla extract (all-natural, sugar-free – or make your own; very easy)
- 1 large (16-ounce) container of organic sour cream
- 1 teaspoon or organic lemon juice (optional)

DIRECTIONS

1. Preheat oven to 350 degrees.
2. Prepare an 8" or 9" springform pan or 9 x 9 pan for cake; or 1 muffin pan.
3. Spray pan with pure avocado or olive oil spray; for muffins, use clean baking cups (such as If You Care Baking Cups)
4. In a large bowl, mix together cream cheese and sweetener.
5. Add vanilla, lemon juice, and sour cream, beating at high speed.
6. Next, add the eggs, one at a time... and beat until well-blended.
7. Spoon/ladle the final mixture into baking pan or baking cups.
8. Bake cake for 40 minutes or muffins for 18-20 minutes.
9. NOTE: Do not overcook; cheesecake will not be firmly set until the cheesecake cools.

BAKING OPTIONS

- Base: We've used ground nuts, crushed low-carb granola, crumbles of low-carb cookies, a package of low-carb graham-cracker crust (1/4 cup), and almond flour (1 cup)... all made by mixing with (1/4 cup) melted butter, a splash of vanilla (and a touch of sweetener if using almond flour)... and then spooning the mixture into the base. If you use a base, bake the base for about 10 minutes prior to adding batter and baking the cheesecake.
- Flavors: We have made chocolate chip, pure chocolate, and pumpkin cheesecake muffins:
- Chocolate Chip: Sprinkle low-carb, no-sugar chocolate chips (such as Lily's) in the batter and/or sprinkle on top prior to baking.
- Chocolate: Mix in up to 1/2 cup unsweetened cocoa powder.
- Pumpkin: Mix in up to one can (15 ounces) of pure pumpkin and 1 tablespoon of pumpkin spice. (Cut back on sour cream for this option.)

Sinfully Delicious Keto, No-Sugar Pecan Pie Muffins

What follows is a very easy recipe for making delicious no-sugar, low-carb pecan pie muffins... perfect for the holidays. It takes about 15 minutes of prep time, and another 15-20 minutes for baking. Makes 12 muffins

INGREDIENTS

- 1 cup butter
- 2/3 cup Swerve (erythritol) brown sugar blend
- 3 eggs
- 2 cups chopped pecans
- 2/3 cup almond flour (or other keto baking mix)

DIRECTIONS

1. Preheat oven to 350F.
2. Place cupcake papers in 2 six-muffin or 1 12-muffin muffin tin.
3. Cream butter, eggs, and Swerve brown sugar.
4. Mix in flour and pecans until well-blended.
5. Fill each muffin cup in muffin tins with batter.
6. Bake for 15 to 20 minutes, until a wooden pick, inserted in the middle, comes out clean.
7. Cool in pan for 10 to 15 minutes, then remove pan and put on a rack to cool. Serve warm.

Optional: *To make these pecan pie muffins even more sinful, consider whipping up some low-carb whipped cream (grassfed/organic heavy cream, a dash of pure vanilla, and powdered erythritol) to serve on top of each muffin!*

Best Keto Delectable Chocolate Chip Cookies

What follows is an easy recipe for making and baking delectable no-sugar, low-carb, keto chocolate chip cookies. It takes about 10 minutes of prep time, and another 10-13 minutes for baking. Makes a batch of about 16 cookies.

INGREDIENTS

- 1/3 cup powdered erythritol (or similar non-sugar sweetener)
- 1/4 cup Swerve brown "sugar" (or similar non-sugar sweetener)
- 1/2 cup grass-fed butter, softened
- 1 teaspoon pure vanilla extract (all-natural, sugar-free – or make your own)
- 2 cups almond flour
- 3/4 cup keto (no-sugar) chocolate chips
- 1/4 teaspoon of baking soda
- 1 organic egg
- OPTIONAL: 3/4 cup chopped nuts of your choice. (We use walnuts, but pecans are good too.)

DIRECTIONS

1. Preheat oven to 325 degrees. Prepare cookie sheet(s) with parchment paper.
2. In large bowl, mix together butter, flour, and baking soda until well blended.
3. Next, mix in vanilla, erythritol, and egg.
4. Finally, fold in the chocolate chips (and walnuts).
5. Using a tablespoon or other kitchen tool, make about 1" balls and place them on the cookie sheet, about an inch apart.
6. Bake for 10-13 minutes, until the cookies brown along the edges.

Best Keto Holiday Sugarless "Sugar" Cookies

What follows is a fun reimagining of traditional holiday cookies – a sugarless sugar cookie that can be baked right from the bowl or refrigerated overnight for using holiday cookie-cutters. It takes about 10 minutes of prep time, and another 11-13 minutes for baking. Makes a batch of about 16 cookies.

INGREDIENTS

- 1/2 cup allulose (or similar non-sugar sweetener)
- 2 teaspoons pure vanilla extract (all-natural, sugar-free – or make your own)
- 1 cup almond flour
- 1/4 cup coconut flour
- 1/2 teaspoon of baking soda
- 1 organic egg
- 2 tablespoons of grassfed butter or coconut oil, melted

DIRECTIONS

1. Preheat oven to 350 degrees. Prepare cookie sheet(s) with parchment paper.
2. In large bowl, mix together dry ingredients until well blended.
3. Next, mix in vanilla and egg to the dry mix.
4. Finally, fold in butter/oil.
5. If making holiday cookie designs, refrigerate dough in covered bowl for several hours or overnight.
6. Otherwise, using a tablespoon or small ice cream scoop, drop rounded balls of dough onto baking sheet.
7. Sprinkle a small amount of allulose crystals or powdered "sugar" on each cookie ball.
8. Bake for 11-13 minutes, until the cookies reach your desired state; bake longer for crispier cookies.

Nutritiously Yummy Sweet Potato Biscuit Cookies

Wonderfully crispy on the outside and chewy on the inside, filled with the amazing nutrients found in sweet potatoes. It takes about 10 minutes of prep time, and another 10-12 minutes for baking. Makes a batch of about 16-20 cookies.

INGREDIENTS

- 1/2 cup cooked and mashed sweet potato
- 2 tablespoons Swerve (or similar non-sugar sweetener)
- 2 teaspoons of cinnamon
- 4 tablespoons grass-fed butter, softened
- 1 teaspoon pure vanilla extract (all-natural, sugar-free – or make your own)
- 2 cups almond flour
- 3 teaspoons of baking powder
- 1 teaspoon of baking soda
- 4 organic eggs

DIRECTIONS

1. Preheat oven to 425 degrees. Prepare large cookie sheet with parchment paper.
2. In large bowl, mix together butter, flour, baking powder, and baking soda until well blended.
3. Add in vanilla, erythritol, and eggs.
4. Next, mix in sweet potato, cinnamon, and Swerve/sweetener.
5. Consistency of batter should be about the same as cookie dough, so adjust flour as needed.
6. Using an ice cream scoop or tablespoon, make about 1" balls and place them on the cookie sheet, about an inch apart.
7. Bake for ten minutes on low rack in over, but check to see at 5 minutes to see if getting too brown. Bake until the outside is brown and crispy.

Optional: You can also try adding nutmeg and switching to Swerve brown "sugar" – or go the savory route and add some onion, garlic, sage to the mix instead of the cinnamon and sweetener.

To add more fluff to your biscuits, you can separate the egg whites and yolks; add the yolks per the recipe, but whip eggs whites separately to stiffness and fold into the batter as a last step before placing on cookie sheet.

Decadent and Simple Baked Pecan Snack

Nuts should be an essential part of your diet for both the fiber and nutrients. Pecans are the perfect nut to make a variety of savory, sweet, or spicy snacks. It takes about 5 minutes of prep time, and another 12-15 minutes for baking.

SALTY PEACAN INGREDIENTS

- 4 cups (32-ounce bag) of raw pecan halves
- 1 stick of grassfed butter, softened
- 2 teaspoons of Himalayan (or other healthy) salt

SAVORY PEACAN INGREDIENTS

- 4 cups (32-ounce bag) of raw pecan halves
- 1 stick of grassfed butter, softened
- 1-2 teaspoons of Himalayan (or other healthy) salt
- 1/2 teaspoon (or more if you love spicy) Cayenne pepper, or similar hot spice

SWEET PEACAN INGREDIENTS

- 4 cups (32-ounce bag) of raw pecan halves
- 1 stick of grassfed butter, softened
- 2 teaspoons of ground cinnamon
- 4 teaspoons of granular allulose, Swerve

DIRECTIONS

1. Preheat oven to 350 degrees.
2. Prepare large cookie sheet (or two smaller ones) with parchment paper.
3. In large bowl, mix together all ingredients except pecans until well blended.
4. Add pecans and keep stirring until all the pecans are coated in mixture.
5. Spread pecans on the cookie sheet, making sure all are flatly on the surface.
6. Before placing in over, consider sprinkling additional salt, spices, or Swerve.
7. Bake for 12 minutes, tossing/flipping pecans about halfway through baking.
8. Remove from oven and let cool; pecans will get firmer/better as they cool.
9. Enjoy for several days, keeping uneaten treats in an airtight container.

Old Fashioned Baked Apples With Kefir

Here's an amazing and healthy twist on your grandmother's baked apple recipe. It's a wonderful treat, and perfect as a delicious and healthy dessert for a chilly fall or winter night. It takes about 25 minutes of prep time, and another 45 minutes for baking.

INGREDIENTS FOR BAKED APPLES

- 6 organic apples, preferably Fuji or Gala
- 1 stick of grassfed butter
- 3 tablespoons ground cinnamon
- 1/2 teaspoon nutmeg
- 1/4 cup stevia or allulose
- 1/4 cup Swerve brown sugar

INGREDIENTS FOR KEFIR TOPPING

- 2 cups of plain, no-sugar Kefir
- 4 tablespoons of stevia or allulose
- 2 teaspoons of ground cinnamon
- 1/2 chopped walnuts

DIRECTIONS

1. Preheat oven to 350 degrees.
2. Core whole apples almost to the bottom, leaving about a half inch; don't cut all the way through.
3. In a small bowl, mix together all the dry ingredients.
4. Place the apples in a 2 to 2.5-qt baking dish.
5. Spoon the brown sugar mixture evenly into the apples.
6. Top each apple with a chunk of butter.
7. Add 1/4 cup of water into bottom of the baking dish.
8. Bake for about 45 minutes, until the apples are tender when pierced with a sharp knife.
9. Take apples out of oven and let cool.
10. In separate bowl, combine Kefir, sweetener, and cinnamon.
11. When apples are still warm, pour the Kefir mix onto the apples, top with walnuts, and serve.

Hydrating and Refreshing Kefir Coconut Drink

Here's an amazingly delicious, nutritious, and refreshing alternative to sugary sodas, juices, and energy drinks that uses only two ingredients, including freeze-dried Kefir starter culture. It takes about 10 minutes of prep time, and another several days for the finished drink. Makes a batch of about 4 glasses/servings.

INGREDIENTS

- 4 cups of coconut water
- 1 packet of Kiefer powder starter (such as Cultures for Health Kefir Starter Culture)

DIRECTIONS

1. Clean and prepare several swing-top bottles that have the locking clamp down caps.
2. In a large bowl, combine the coconut water and powdered cultures.
3. Stir thoroughly until powder completely dissolved.
4. Pour into bottles, leaving at least 1 inch of space at the top.
5. Clamp the caps and put aside in an area with no direct sunlight, for 2-3 days.
6. Check bottles and once they have enough bubbles for your liking, place in refrigerator.

NOTES:

- Sealed bottles can be stored in the refrigerator for about three weeks.
- Keep bottles sealed until use, otherwise carbonation will decrease rapidly.
- Try adding flavors to your drinks, such as adding a half cup of fruit extract, such as lemon, lime, strawberry, cherry, or tangerine. Or, make it spicy with by adding some herbs, such as ginger.
- Switch out the coconut water (or some of it) with juice as a base, such as: watermelon, grapes, oranges, sweet lime, and grapefruit.

Easy, Healthy, and Organic Vanilla Extract

Stop buying cheap imitation vanilla or expensive organic vanilla extract by making your own. It's simple to do, a healthy and cheaper alternative, and it makes a great gift to other bakers. It takes about 10 minutes of prep time, and another six+ months for the finished (best) product. Makes a batch of about 4 glasses/servings.

INGREDIENTS

- 2 cups of organic Vodka (I use Akva Organic Swedish Vodka)
- 6-8 vanilla bean pods (Madagascar Vanilla Beans Grade A or Grade B)

DIRECTIONS

1. Prepare one or two tall bottles with swing-top or screw cap. (Amber bottles work best.)
2. Cut vanilla pods down the center.
3. Fill bottle(s) with vodka, enough to cover the vanilla pods.
4. Place vanilla pods in bottle(s) with vodka.
5. Seal bottle(s) and place in a dark, cool cupboard.
6. Every few weeks, flip the bottle.
7. For every week/month of sitting, the vanilla will get darker, richer.

CHAPTER ELEVEN
Top Tips from Expert Nutritionists/Dietitians

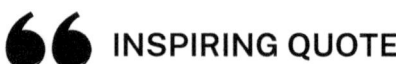

INSPIRING QUOTE

"The primary reason diseases tend to run in families may be that diets tend to run in families." — Michael Greger

No one holds the wisdom for any subject; it truly takes a community.

Thus, I invited some of my favorite doctors, nutrients, and dietitians to submit their best nutrition tip. If a tip resonates with you, I encourage you to then connect and follow these experts; some are also coaches who may be able to provide additional support for you as you make the transition from poor foods and diets to better ones.

HERE ARE THE EXPERT TIPS!

HEALTHY EATING MEANS DIFFERENT THINGS TO DIFFERENT PEOPLE.

What is universal is the idea that if you eat non-processed foods, with minimal additives and no artificial ingredients, you will be better off. It is best to eat lots of fruit, vegetables, and protein from whatever source you prefer. Meat, fish, chicken, and plant-based sources are all fine as long as you eat a varied diet filled with color, variety, and love. We all know that wholesome foods beat out processed foods every time, but it is also important to enjoy your food and enjoy your life.

One of the best ways to enjoy your food and optimize your health is to slow down, eat slowly, and chew your food with at least 20 chews before you swallow.

Eat with others whenever possible so you don't experience loneliness, and make mealtime a main event rather than an afterthought in your day.

-PATRICIA GREENBERG, chef and fitness expert, passionate pro-aging advocate, dedicated to promoting wellness and longevity.
WEBSITE: patriciagreenberg.com/
FACEBOOK: https://www.facebook.com/patricia.greenberg.14

SO MANY PEOPLE GET STUCK IN A RUT EATING THE SAME THINGS OVER AND OVER AGAIN.

However, lack of diversity in our diets leads to a less diverse gut microbiome and increases the possibility of dysbiosis and all the negative health consequences that come along with it. My challenge to all of my clients is to eat the most diverse diet possible, depending on their stage of healing.

When in the grocery store, choose one new fruit or vegetable to try each week to slowly work on building diversity in your diet. You can involve the whole family and even make a game out of it, seeing who can find something new each week!

-REBECCA ARSENA, Certified Functional Nutrition Counselor, NBC-HWC, Functional Medicine Certified Health Coach
WEBSITE: rebeccaarsena.com | INSTAGRAM: @rebeccaarsena
EMAIL: info@rebeccaarsena.com

IF YOU CRAVE PROCESSED OR FAST FOOD OVER MORE NOURISHING OPTIONS, KNOW THAT THIS ISN'T ACCIDENTAL.

Food companies deliberately create irresistible, addictive products that hijack your brain chemically for their profit. Your preferences are a result of this manipulated food environment. Multiple factors contribute to your eating behaviors: genetics, family history, and household rules. Childhood experiences, like ice cream dates with a grandparent, can create lasting positive associations. Guilt-inducing messages like "Clean your plate!" can also play a role.

We eat for celebration and eat more when those around us eat more. Stress and trauma can impact eating, as can challenges in recognizing our own emotions and unmet needs. Misleading media and food marketing exacerbate these struggles.

Shame has no place around eating. While change can be hard, it's possible (and maybe enjoyable!) with support. Don't hesitate to seek help – you don't have to figure it out alone.

-JANET FRANK, PH.D., NBC-HWC, A-CFHC, PFAC,
National Board Certified Health and Wellness Coach, ADAPT Certified Functional Health Coach, Professional Food Addiction Coach
LINKEDIN: linkedin.com/in/janetfrankphdnbchwc/ | WEBSITE: JanetFrankCoaching.com
EMAIL: janetfrankcoaching@gmail.com

IN TODAY'S HECTIC WORLD, FAMILY MEALS PLAY A CRUCIAL ROLE IN OUR HEALTH AND WELL-BEING.

As a former educator turned nutrition advocate, I've seen how prioritizing family mealtime can enhance children's health, academic performance, and overall family wellness.

Making family meals a daily ritual is linked to improved digestion, better gut health, and a reduced risk of chronic illness. Introducing vegetables to babies early helps develop a natural craving for healthy foods.

Involving children in meal preparation promotes healthy eating habits. With 1 in 6 U.S. kids struggling with obesity, these habits are crucial for prevention.

Beyond nourishment, family meals strengthen bonds, support academic success, and instill lifelong healthy habits. Creating a positive, stress-free dining environment enhances emotionalwell-being.

Embrace family meals to nurture our bodies, minds, and hearts, making mealtime a cornerstone of holistic health.

-TAMMIE MATTOS, Certified Health Coach & Family Nutrition Advocate
WEBSITE: tammiemattos.com/ | LINKEDIN: linkedin.com/in/tammie-mattos
EMAIL: tammiemattos@gmail.com

NEVER LOSE SIGHT OF HOW AMAZING YOUR BODY IS IN HEALING ITSELF!

From diet and food to mental health and physical ailments, your body is constantly healing and adapting. Always remember that your body is made of energy.

By learning to heal energetically, you CAN control the future of your health in preventative care as well as reversing mental belief or heart-brain cohesion disconnection (which is cause to many issues) in order to achieve your true purpose, freedom, and joy here on earth. To work with your body (aka energy), you must start with your HEART.

Touch your heart right now and say "I love you." Feel the loving vibrations and do this every day. When YOU heal, you heal those you love, and affect the world.

-JANLIA RILEY, CECP, CBCP, BCP3
WEBSITE: HeartfulLiving.today | INSTAGRAM/FACEBOOK: @heartfullivingtoday
EMAIL: smile@heartfulliving.today

INCORPORATE FRUITS AND VEGETABLES INTO EVERY MEAL!

Don't just add them as sides, but INFUSE THEM into everything. If you drink water, put orange, cucumber, or strawberries into it. If you make a smoothie of any fruit, always add a giant handful of spinach.

If you make salads, chop up apples and toss in blueberries. Love Italian food, make your own noodles and blend spinach and carrots into the dough (whole wheat that is!). Peanut butter on toast fan? Slice up an apple or banana and put on top.

Waffles can actually be made from sweet potatoes, and noodles can be spiralized from zucchini and sauteed like pasta, you could add homemade tomato sauce with minced mushrooms like a Bolognese.

Fruits and vegetables give you fiber, phytochemicals, vitamins and minerals, improve your immunity, help you maintain a healthy weight, and lead you toward long term health free of chronic disease.

-MANDY RODRIGUES, ED.D.
WEBSITE: https://empowertunity.com/
LINKEDIN: linkedin.com/in/mandy-rodrigues/

LIFE SHAPES AND MOLDS US, WHETHER POSITIVELY OR NEGATIVELY; THESE EXPERIENCES SHAPE HOW WE VIEW FOOD, FLUIDS, MOVEMENT, SLEEP, AND STRESS MANAGEMENT, WHILE DIET CULTURE IN OUR SOCIETY ALSO TELLS US OUR BODIES DETERMINE OUR SELF-WORTH.

The truth is, there isn't a "one size fits all" for our individual needs, including our health and wellness journey. As a Doctor of Clinical Nutrition, Certified Nutrition Specialist, and Licensed Dietitian Nutritionist, it's about giving yourself permission because this isn't about willpower but motivation on what makes you feel good and will lessen your root cause for making the changes.

Teaching yourself to eat, drink, move, sleep, and manage your stress in a way that feels good to you and resonates with your lifestyle with slow, small, and steady steps will allow you to encompass healthy changes that are sustainable for the long haul.

-DR LINNETTE M. JOHNSON, DCN, CNS,
Licensed Dietitian and Owner at 5 Elements Coaching
WEBSITE: 5elementscoaching.org | INSTAGRAM: @5elementswellnesscenter
EMAIL: info@5elementscoaching.org

ONE TIP FOR THOSE SUFFERING FROM TYPE 2 DIABETES IS TO ACTUALLY WITHHOLD FROM EATING IN THE FORM OF HEALTHY INTERMITTENT FASTING.

New research is showing that people have put their Type 2 Diabetes into remission by fasting 16 hours – and then eating within an 8-hour time frame during the day.

One other tip for helping combat Type 2 Diabetes is for people to consume mushrooms on a regular basis. Reshi, Maitake, Shiitake, Lion's Mane, and Cordyceps mushrooms have all been shown to lower blood sugar levels for Type II Diabetics. Matter of fact, mushrooms are a brilliant choice for anyone's optimal health!

-JANELLE CWIK, **Certified Life & Health Coach at Twin Lions Global Health**
WEBSITE: twinlionsgh.com
LINKEDIN: linkedin.com/in/janelle-marlie-lysbeth-cwik-727a88151/
EMAIL: energymaster217@gmail.com

CANDIDA IS A NATURALLY OCCURRING FUNGUS THAT LIVES IN OUR BODIES, HOWEVER, WHEN AN OVERGROWTH OCCURS, IT TURNS INTO A DANGEROUS YEAST (CANDIDIASIS).

Fed mainly by excessive sugar and stress, this out of balance pest can negatively impact our health in myriad ways and eventually get into our bloodstream. A simple way to check your body is by performing "the spit test."

First thing in the morning, fill a clear glass halfway to the top with water, then spit into it! Ideally, your spit will float on top of the water, but if after 30-45 minutes it looks like a jellyfish from the side with long stringy legs, or you see cloudy floating specks, it is highly likely that you have a Candida overgrowth. Not to worry, as this is manageable by eating a 21-day elimination diet to starve the yeast of the sugar that feeds it, allowing your body to come back into balance more readily.

-JAYNE BAKER, CNHP, President of Momentum Lifestyle Consulting
WEBSITE: momentumlifestyleconsulting.com
INSTAGRAM: @BreakYourInertia
FACEBOOK: facebook.com/BreakYourInertia

TO EFFECTIVELY MANAGE IBS, ADOPT A HOLISTIC APPROACH THAT INTEGRATES DIET, MOVEMENT, STRESS MANAGEMENT, AND ADEQUATE REST.

Prioritize whole foods that support gut health, including fiber-rich fruits, vegetables, whole grains, and lean proteins. These nourish your microbiome and promote healthy digestion. Complement your diet with regular movement; gentle exercises like walking, yoga, and stretching can aid digestion and reduce stress.

Manage stress through mindfulness practices such as meditation, deep breathing, and positive thinking to minimize IBS flare-ups. Ensure you get sufficient rest and quality sleep, as they are crucial for gut health and overall well-being. By combining these elements, you create a balanced lifestyle that supports gut health and helps manage IBS symptoms more effectively. Remember, a healthy gut is integral to your overall health and vitality.

-MARICA GASPIC PISKOVIC, B.SC.PHM,
Pharmacist, Certified Holistic Health and Wellness Coach
WEBSITE: www.gutwellnessbymarica.com
INSTAGRAM: @gutwellnessbymarica

BONUS TIPS FROM NUTRITION GURUS!

THE BEST THING YOU CAN DO FOR YOUR HEALTH IS TO COOK YOUR OWN FOOD.

You save money. You get healthier. You feel better. You look better.

This is the way.

–DR. JAMES DINICOLANTONIO, Doctor of Pharmacy

WEBSITE: drjamesdinic.com | INSTAGRAM: @drjamesdinic

BOOK: *The Obesity Fix: How to Beat Food Cravings, Lose Weight and Gain Energy*

EVERYTHING IS IMPORTANT... UNTIL YOU'RE SICK.

Then only one thing is important... your health.

Yet you consistently sacrifice your health for things that aren't all that important.

Invest daily into maintaining and improving your health so that you can give 100 percent to all of the things in your life that actually matter.

–DR. CALEB BURGESS DPT OCS CSCS

INSTAGRAM: dr.caleb.burgess

THERE IS ONE INGREDIENT THAT'S SO COMMON IN PROCESSED FOODS THAT ALMOST EVERYONE EATS IT DAILY.

The average American consumes 38 pounds of it yearly.

This ingredient is Soybean Oil.

And it has a detrimental effect on our health.

–VANI HARI: THE FOOD BABE

WEBSITE: FOODBABE.COM/ | INSTAGRAM: @THEFOODBABE

BOOK: *Feeding You Lies: How to Unravel the Food Industry's Playbook and Reclaim Your Health*

AS EXPENSIVE AS IT IS TO EAT HEALTHY FOOD, IT IS EVEN MORE EXPENSIVE TO HAVE OBESITY, DIABETES, HEART DISEASE, OR ALZHEIMER'S DISEASE.

-ROBERT LUFKIN, MD, metabolic health and longevity expert

WEBSITE: robertlufkinmd.com | INSTAGRAM: @robertlufkinmd

BOOK: *Lies I Taught in Medical School: How Conventional Medicine Is Making You Sicker and What You Can Do to Save Your Own Life Health*

EAT PLENTY OF NATURAL PLANTS AND ANIMALS: UNCANNED, UNPROCESSED, AND ORGANIC, IF POSSIBLE.

Eat real, whole foods. You will avoid many common illnesses by simply eating natural, whole foods. The closer it is to the earth or sea from which it came, the more whole it is.

Rethink your priorities. A shopping bag full of healthy food may cost you a few bucks more. But if you had a serious illness, you'd pay any price to be healed. You will pay a big price for eating the emp[ty calories of junk food. Think of the extra cost now as an investment in fabulous health.

-DR. FRANK KING, naturopath and chiropractor

WEBSITE: drkings.com/

BOOK: *The Healing Revolution: Eight Essential to Awaken Abundant Life, Naturally!*

PART THREE: HEALTH, NUTRITION, AND DIET SUCCESS STORIES

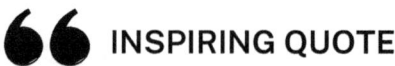 **INSPIRING QUOTE**

"Fitness is 20% exercise and 80% nutrition. You can't outrun your fork." — Unknown

CHAPTER TWELVE
David's Story

SO, WHO THE HECK IS DAVID MEDANSKY AND WHY SHOULD YOU LISTEN TO HIM?

Name: David Medansky

How do you feel (mentally and physically) now? Awesome!

How were you (mentally and physically) before you started? Embarrassed, frustrated, tired.

Best aspect of your plan: Simple to do.

Hardest part of your plan: Doing what we know we can do because it's not what we can it's what we WILL do.

Key indicators of your health and healing: More energy, weight-loss, no afternoon brain fog, better mental clarity, improved overall health, feel and look better.

Biggest surprise of your health journey: Enjoying my new lifestyle and healthy eating habits.

Maybe you are like me; we were fit and trim when we were younger. However, as with most people, life gets in the way, whether it be family or work obligations. Maybe you, like me, stopped exercising. Or, like me, you started eating more fast food and convenience foods.

Instead of eating one scoop of ice cream, I'd eat an entire pint in one sitting. Or an entire canister of Pringles. If there was a special buy-one-get-one-free sandwich at a fast-food place, I'd eat both sandwiches. I was disgusted with myself. I couldn't believe my pants size ballooned up.

Perhaps, like me, the weight crept up on you.

Like you, I struggled with weight issues and dieting. I went on many different diets, looking for the perfect one. However, no matter what I did or what diet I attempted, I failed.

If I did lose weight, I wasn't able to keep it off.

Then something happened to turn my life around. I dubbed it my wake-up call.

In July 2016, at age 61, my doctor told me that based on my lab results and being fat, I had a 95 percent chance of having a fatal heart attack. He gave me two options: 1) lose weight, or 2) find a new doctor because he did not want me to die on his watch. In most things, I am pleased to be in the 95th percentile. However, its different if it meant I was likely to die.

Suddenly, my being fat was more than just embarrassing, it was lethal.

With that sword hanging over my head, I managed to shed 50 pounds over the next four months, nearly a quarter of my total body weight. More importantly, I have kept the weight off since then. Now I feel great, I have more energy, better mental clarity, and I have improved my overall health.

I learned how to lose weight without going on a diet, without exercising, without counting calories, and without needing to buy any special meals, supplements, or products. I did a tremendous amount of research on the subject. This much I know: when it comes to losing weight, keeping it off, and living a healthy life, it's not one size fits all.

Six years after getting that scary diagnosis, in June of 2022, at age 67, I hiked Mt. Kilimanjaro.

I think most people know what to do to eat healthy; they just don't do it. Why? Why is it so difficult to live a healthy lifestyle? Probably because it's not what we can do, rather, it's what we *will* do. And that's the answer – knowing what you can do, yet not *willing* to do it.

After I released my unwanted and unhealthy weight, I started rereading the health books I read in the 1970s, such as *Sugar Blues* by William Dufty, books by Paul and Patricia Bragg, Jack LaLanne, Richard Simmons, and others to improve my eating habits and overall health.

Being a former lawyer, I am trained to do research. To sift through information and discern between fact, opinion, and fiction. While doing my research for healthy weight-loss, I was overwhelmed and inundated with the amount of information available. Thousands and thousands of books have been written about diet, nutrition, fitness, and exercise.

Right now, there are more than 50,000 books available on Amazon pertaining to diet, weight-loss, health, fitness, and nutrition. At the grocery store checkout, you'll see hundreds of magazine articles written about health and wellness. Thousands of blogs and articles are available when you search online as well as videos on YouTube. Numerous weight-loss programs, both national and local, are advertised on TV, radio, and social media.

With all the information out there about health, wellness, and nutrition, who or what do you believe and act on? How do you choose? One expert will tell you one thing; another will say exactly the opposite. A third expert will then tell you the other two are wrong.

As a lawyer, I spent my career seeing both sides of the fence – honest people and dishonest people. And when it comes to the food, pharmaceutical, and weight-loss industries, sadly, there are more dishonest people than there are those telling the truth. That's what makes living a healthy lifestyle so difficult. My friend Michaela Gaffen Stone said, "The food companies will get you sick, Big Pharma will keep you sick, and the diet and weight loss industries are aiding and abetting both of them."

Just like I had to read the fine print when I practiced law, I am now reading the fine print on food labels. Consider this: if weight-loss and diet programs worked, we'd all be thinner and healthier, and those companies would be out of business after a few years. They depend on repeat customers to stay relevant. When I started my health journey in 2016, diet and weight loss was a $62 billion per year industry. Today, it's more than $82 Billion. In other words, we are getting fatter.

The average person will attempt four to five new diets each year. During a lifetime, a person will attempt, on average, 126 different diets. What this means for you is that diets don't work. Rather than going on a diet that is temporary, extreme, hard to stick to, and potentially dangerous to your health, change your lifestyle and eating habits.

You will never improve your health until you change your daily eating habits and routines. The secret of you living a healthy lifestyle is found in your daily eating practices. A routine becomes a behavior. Behavior becomes a habit. And a habit is something you just do.

According to Cardiologist, Dr. Mimi Guarneri, "70 to 90 percent of chronic diseases is related to lifestyle and environment. Where you live, who you live with, what you eat, are you breathing clean air, are you drinking filtered clean water, what king of toxins are in your life, and so on."

Research also shows that 90 to 95 percent of your body weight and shape is determined by your diet, what you eat and drink, and only 5 to 10 percent is determined by your physical activity and other factors such as hormones or medical conditions. People always confuse exercising with weight-loss. You can shed weight without exercising. However, you can never exercise enough to overcome poor eating habits.

Isn't that right, Bob Harper of *The Biggest Loser* fame?

In early 2017, Bob Harper had a heart attack at the gym during his workout. He was only 52 years old. Being one of the biggest names in the fitness industry, Harper's heart attack came as a shock since many people believed he depicted excellent health.

After his heart attack, Harper made lifestyle changes to become healthier. He says, "I've been in the health and fitness industry for almost 30 years now, but I had to pivot my life and redefine the way that I ate and worked out." Now he primarily follows a Mediterranean diet.

Exercise is not the best way to lose weight. Exercising to lose weight is a myth. Here is why. Most people overestimate how many calories they burn during a workout and underestimate how many calories they consume. Plus, most people tend to eat more when they exercise because they're hungrier.

Fat and muscle weigh the same. Five pounds of fat weighs the same as five pounds of muscle. However, fat takes up more space than muscle. When you burn fat and increase muscle mass, you either won't lose weight or you will gain weight. Would this frustrate you if you put in the hours of exercising thinking you are losing weight only to see the scale read the same or more? For most people it becomes extremely discouraging, and they quit.

Many people set expectations about the number on the scale, and when those expectations are not met, they quit, they give up. This might explain why people who make New Year's resolutions to exercise and lose weight stop after a few weeks. Many fail to keep up their workouts because they are not seeing immediate results. Or, their new exercise schedule and routine is not conducive to their family obligations, work responsibilities, and lifestyle.

It is not about the number on the scale, it is about the inches of your waistline.

Exercise, however, is important for being fit and for overall health and wellness. Once you shed many of your extra pounds you will most likely want to be more physically active and begin an exercise program.

Thomas Edison said, "The doctor of the future will give no medicine but will interest his patients in the care of the human frame, in diet and in the cause and prevention of disease." Edison was wrong. The future is now, yet we consume more highly processed and manufactured foods that are scientifically engineered and full of chemicals. These foods are addictive and deadly.

Furthermore, technology allows us to do fewer physical activities, i.e., not getting off the couch to change the TV channel because we have remote controls, spending more time on computers and watching TV than playing outside, and the political climate which limits children from playing outdoors and having physical education classes.

More people are taking medications for preventable diseases and ailments. It's the new normal. I challenge you to be the exception. It's not about my being right or wrong. It's about what you will do. Will you be a part of the new normal or dare to be different?

So, you might be wondering what can I do to live a healthier life? After thousands of hours of research, in my opinion, it comes down to 9 simple rules.

MY GOLDEN RULES FOR A HEALTHIER LIFE

1. Drink more pure water (distilled, high quality reputable source Spring water, or six stage reverse osmosis filtering system). Drink at least one-half of your total body weight in ounces of water. For example, if you weigh 200 pounds, drink 100 ounces of water.
2. Avoid highly processed, ultra processed, and manufactured foods.
3. Eat real, whole, holistic foods (vegetables, fruits, berries, nuts, legumes).
4. Eat slower.
5. Eat smaller portions. Use a salad plate instead of a dinner plate.
6. Get 7 to 8 hours of quality sleep.
7. Rest to digest. That's a 12-hour intermittent fast. The easiest way to accomplish this is to stop eating three hours before you go to sleep, sleep for 7 to 8 hours, and have your first meal 2 to 3 hours after you wake up. That's it. Most people do it without realizing it. When you first wake up drink a minimum of eight ounces of water. This will rehydrate you and water is a natural appetite suppressant.
8. Think positively. Eighty percent of our thoughts are negative. Imagine if we reversed it to eighty percent positive.
9. Walk each day a minimum of 30 minutes. You do not need to walk the thirty minutes all at one time. You can break it up into two or three shorter walks throughout the day.

These are simple everyday things that you CAN do. Don't let the simplicity of these rules fool you – they are game changers.

I am not a doctor. Nor am I a mental or health professional. However, I understand the challenges, frustrations, and obstacles people will face along the journey to living a healthy lifestyle.

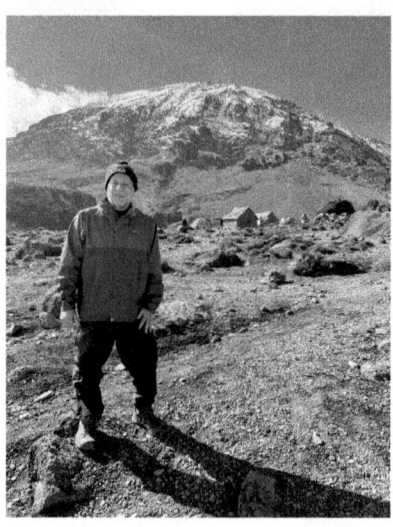

David Medansky, during his hike of Mt. Kilimanjaro.

David Medansky, award winning, best-selling author, is known as "The Health Guy" because he consults with companies that have between 50 and 150 employees to reduce employee stress, burnout, absenteeism, turnover, and lower health care costs through a result-oriented interactive health and wellness program that empowers CEOs, Executives, and Employees to live a healthy life. David understands your frustrations, embarrassment, and humiliation being overweight, because he too was once fat, unhealthy, and out of shape. Like many of you he attempted countless diets only to be disappointed or frustrated with the results until he learned to change his diet instead of going on a diet.

Learn more at JadedHealth.com (https://www.linkedin.com/in/davidmedansky-the-healthguy/)

EDITOR'S NOTES: KEY TAKEAWAYS FROM DAVID'S STORY

- Do not wait until your doctor gives you a death sentence to start living healthier, eating better, nutrient-dense foods.
- Food companies, Big Pharma, and the diet industry want people confused about nutrition and diet so that people continue to buy more pills and programs.
- Changing diet is essential and life-enhancing. Exercise is important (especially for mental health and longevity), but exercise alone will not heal you/make you healthy.
- Throw away the scale and stop obsessing over your weight. Instead, focus on steady, incremental changes to your diet and lifestyle that improve your health and healing.

CHAPTER THIRTEEN
Jake's Story

SURVIVING TO THRIVING

Name: Jacob Gray

How do you feel (mentally and physically) now? I currently feel better than I ever have before – mentally, physically, and spiritually.

How were you (mentally and physically) before you started? Before I started I was at my lowest ever adult weight, anxious, depressed, angry, and didn't have much be proud of or live for.

Best aspect of your plan: Improving small things over time, 1% better every day.

Hardest part of your plan: I do miss things like pizza and sweets, or going out with friends and having a couple beers. But I'm happier and feel so much better by sticking with my diet and routines.

Key indicators of your health and healing: More energy, amazing restful sleep, mental clarity, no brain fog, no dizziness, less anxiety, no depression, feeling and looking strong and healthy, and better relationships with myself and others.

Biggest surprise of your health journey: How much better I feel all the time, and not realizing it was possible to feel this great again. Also how much diet and lifestyle changes have improved my brain injury symptoms.

My name is Jacob (Jake) Gray. I was born and currently reside in Coeur d' Alene, Idaho. I am 34 years old and a medically retired combat veteran.

I'm currently in the best shape of my life and living a more conscious and healthier lifestyle than I ever have before.

My health journey began in late 2021, but for more context, I'll have to go back a little a bit.

As a kid, my family didn't have much knowledge or interest in healthy eating habits. We weren't in a great place financially and since both my parents worked full time, meals were often whatever was cheapest and easiest. We had lots of frozen pizza, cheap snacks, Kool-Aid, and sodas.

We never had much knowledge or interest into what was the healthiest choice, and that continued through my teen years as well, eating whatever I felt like and wanted. I ate lots of fast food, junk food, sodas, and Gatorade.

The first time I started to think about healthier options was when I started taking racing motocross more seriously so I made efforts to drink more water and maybe choose Subway over Taco Bell. Still not great choices but at least a start.

Unfortunately, while racing I sustained a number of injuries, but the most noteworthy would be having four concussions.

At the time I didn't think the concussions were that significant, but I would later find out that was probably not true.

Then at 19, I joined the Marine Corps as a combat engineer. I was involved in a lot of explosives for training such as cratering, breaching, and mine-clearing.

I deployed to the Helmand province, Afghanistan, in 2009, where my main job was doing route clearance, so basically patrolling in vehicles or on foot searching for IED's (Improvised Explosive Devices).

While conducting route clearance operations, I was directly involved in three IED blasts and received multiple traumatic brain injuries and PTSD as a result. That deployment and the injuries incurred led to me being medically retired in 2013, and that's when my health began to decline.

I returned home to Idaho and began integrating back into my old life, but it didn't take long for things to unravel. I had trouble sleeping, along with memory and attention difficulties, anxiety, depression, irritability, dizziness, and lots of headaches.

I was still being seen through the VA but not getting any noticeable improvement. I tried going the medication route but I had heard a lot of horror stories and never felt like they helped so I didn't continue medication for long.

I also was not taking great care of myself. I had stopped exercising, was eating junk foods constantly, drinking alcohol, and abusing cannabis… just to be able to get to sleep overnight.

I had also gotten down to my lowest ever adult weight of 147 lbs. – and was essentially a shell of myself both physically and mentally.

Things continued to worsen until 2021, when I found out about and got involved with Heroic Hearts Project. I attended an ayahuasca retreat with in Peru in September 2021, which was incredibly beneficial and was the catalyst for me turning my life around. I was able to work through a lot of my traumas from military and childhood and be able to see the repercussions of the lifestyle choices I was making and where that path was leading.

Before consuming the ayahuasca, I had been on a required "dieta." This diet was helpful and was a good cleanse for my body. It's a very minimal diet, focused on plant-based foods free of fats and salts. I would say that doing the initial diet was another catalyst for the start of my healthy lifestyle.

The diet was what made me finally stop daily cannabis use. I now only use it consciously and sparingly. I also don't eat much pork with the diet. It's not a religious thing, but mainly that pork is not the best animal to eat – and they are often fed poor diets to begin with.

I also tend to avoid chicken as most chicken is fed corn and soy, which I avoid, and they do not digest those very well either. The local eggs I buy are corn and soy free. I will only have chicken occasionally.

As soon as I returned from Peru I felt incredible and was reinvigorated with motivation again. I began exercising daily, stopped alcohol and cannabis, starting eating healthy, making sleep a priority, and really began to transform all aspects of my life for the better.

I was then recommended by other vets with head injuries to get my hormones tested, and it turned out I was also dealing with very low testosterone and began testosterone replacement therapy. The third major change began after getting involved in a jiu jitsu gym. Starting jiu jitsu helped me find community that I was missing as well as keeping me accountable for taking care of my health.

Now in 2024, I am living the best and healthiest lifestyle I ever have.

I have seen the impact that making the right decisions can have on mental and physical health and I now make it a priority. I cook all my meals fresh at home.

My current diet is mostly a carnivore and keto based diet and I also drink raw milk and use raw local honey. I will have some fruit from time to time but not daily. I avoid all processed foods, anything with added sugars and seed oils.

It has been a few years since I've eaten any fast food or any kind of junk or unhealthy food. I'm quite consistent with my diet now and my daily meals are almost exactly the same from day to day. My first meal is around 2-3 pm and is four eggs with about a third of a pound of flat steak with cheese, sour cream, a little hot sauce, and raw milk.

I should also add that I try to drink about 30+ ounces of water in the morning before my first meal and more if it's a jiu jitsu day. I even add a pure salt and mineral liquids to my water every time I fill my bottle.

My next meal is around 6-7 pm – and for the last few years, my main meal that I eat almost every day is smoked tri-tip beef. I have about one pound or slightly less and use a homemade seasoning, then smoke it for about an hour, and pan sear it in a cast iron. I only cook in stainless or cast iron, never any non-stick pans. I use wood cutting boards and avoid plastics whenever possible.

I source my food locally as much as I can. My eggs, honey, and raw milk come from an hour away, the meat comes from southern Idaho. The only things I don't get locally right now are sour cream, cheese, and hot sauce. I only shop at a local health food store named Pilgrims and only eat organic foods.

I rarely drink alcohol anymore; maybe on special occasions.

I prioritize staying hydrated and even use a stainless steel gravity water filter the eliminates as much toxins as possible. I built my own cold plunge out of an old ice chest. I have my own weights at home so not only do I go to jiu jitsu 5-6 days a week for two hours a day but also try to lift weights 4-5 times a week as well.

I do yoga and mobility work every morning and every night before bed. I intermittent fast, so my first meal of the day is around 2-3pm and dinner around 7pm.

I also read for 30 minutes before bed overnight and prioritize a healthy sleep routine.

Not only through my own journey, but also through watching other people – including my family – I have been able to get an in-depth perspective about the impact food and lifestyle choices can have. My father has dealt with ulcerative colitis and Crohn's disease for 8 years and even had a stroke in 2022. As much as my mother and I have tried to help him, he has always believed that there is a pill to fix everything and hasn't taken full responsibility and accountability for his life and choices.

Seeing my father's struggles, as well as having my own, it has become abundantly clear how important it is to take full control over one's own health.

It has become very clear to me over the years that you can't rely on doctors or modern medicine to always have the answers or know what's best for you. You need to do your own research and be your own advocate.

Along with diet, exercise, and lifestyle changes, I have a deep relationship with plant medicines – and they have been hugely beneficial for my mental and even physical health. They were the catalyst that started me on healthier living.

Because of this, I now am an ambassador and veteran liaison for Heroic Hearts Project, and am committed to helping other veterans find peace and get their lives back as well. I will be returning to Peru with another group of veterans this fall and hope to help others on their journey.

In conclusion, the advice I would have for anyone getting started in a healthier lifestyle is to not get overwhelmed at first… and start small. A great book I read recently called *Atomic Habits* goes into detail about how to make habit changes and how to make them stick; one of the biggest lessons I got was to make small changes over time. Start with one thing, and once that thing becomes a habit, then add in another healthy choice and so on. Oftentimes, people will dive into the deep end and try to change too much too soon and it becomes too difficult to stick to those changes.

Also, be more in the mindset of the grocery store being your pharmacy. You can heal so many things by eating healthy and making some other healthy habit changes like daily movement.

The last thing I would recommend is to do your own research on what's actually healthy or not; you can't always listen to the experts. In the 1960's, the sugar research foundation paid Harvard scientists the equivalent of $50,000 in today's money to publish a review of research to point the finger for heart disease at fat instead of sugar. It's now known that healthy fats are a crucial part of our diet, so you can't always believe what you're told; you have to learn for yourself.

Jacob Gray lives in North Idaho, is a veteran liaison for Heroic Hearts Project, and also has a wellness and plant medicine mentoring business: Micromind Wellness. You can find him on Instagram @gsd_132 or @micromindwellness.

EDITOR'S NOTES: KEY TAKEAWAYS FROM JAKE'S STORY

- Many of us learn our bad eating habits during childhood – consuming too many sweets, sodas, chips, and fast foods – but as adults we need to break free of those childhood habits that no longer work for us by focusing on heathy eating that will help us live better lives.
- Concussions and brain injuries can cause long-lasting and negative health effects unless treated properly. If you have suffered one or more, seek out restorative treatments like Jake.

- Remember that healing and health are multifaceted and that you may need to take several different approaches on your journey to find your optimal health and healing.
- It may seem hard to believe, but simply changing your diet to healthy foods will result in dramatic shifts in health and well-being.
- Partaking in a healing journey, especially when plant medicines are used as a tool, often propels and motivates people to seek healthy habits and lifestyles.

CHAPTER FOURTEEN
Kali's Story

INTEGRATION AND DIET

Name: Kali Archipley, AE1(AW), USN–R

How do you feel (mentally and physically) now? Very well regulated, clear, healthy.

How were you (mentally and physically) before you started? Tired, depressed, suicidal.

Best aspect of your plan: Modular, intuitive, creative.

Hardest part of your plan: Sitting in discomfort of emotions, breaking away from cultural standards.

Key indicators of your health and healing: Reduction in symptoms of PTSD, depression. Weight and hormone regulation.

Biggest surprise of your health journey: How vastly different it is from where I was before, and how much my perspective on food and society has shifted in the process.

It's hard for me to pinpoint where the beginning of my healing journey started. My first answer would be 2022, when I started microdosing and really analyzing myself and my mental health in relation to my environment. But wounds begin the process of healing as soon as the trauma occurs, so in reality, my healing journey began in 2012… or maybe even at birth. *We all have something to heal from.*

I enlisted in the U.S. Navy in 2011, as an Aviation Electrician's Mate, and excelled to the rank of E–6 in 5 years, in spite of many hurdles. I served ten years, spending time in Hawaii, Sicily, Guam, Japan, and several locations stateside.

During my time in service, I experienced three separate military sexual traumas, which ultimately led me to be medically retired in 2020 for PTSD. My symptoms had gotten so severe; I existed with chronic suicidal ideation, anxiety, and depression that I could no longer hide or manage. I spent more than 100 days inpatient during my career, had been prescribed about a dozen different pharmaceuticals, and somehow ended up with close to 20 separate diagnoses in my medical record.

The Navy holds high standards for its servicemembers' body composition. Because of this, I struggled with diet and weight loss my whole career, even though I was never technically overweight. I can see now that I had developed a mild case of Orthorexia. I was obsessed with counting macros, protein, and measuring myself. I would do extreme water fasts to cut weight and experimented with supplements to enhance weight loss and performance. I started lifting and competing as a powerlifter, and I was pretty good at it. People often came to me for advice, and I ended up working to become a certified personal trainer.

When I left the military, I was terrified but hopeful for the future. When I received my separation papers, I was 7 months pregnant with my twin sons during the height of the COVID–19 pandemic. It was incredibly lonely and scary, and definitely did not lend well to my mental health.

Bringing home our newborns was the first time I was forced to shift my perspective away from my powerlifting/military style diet. I had gained 60 pounds carrying my boys, and I had to work really hard to reduce the amount of anxiety and shame I carried within my postpartum body. I learned everything I could about how to increase and sustain lactation, which, surprise, doesn't actually involve eating cookies loaded with fenugreek. (Supplements are unregulated and many sold for lactation support are potentially harmful to babies.)

It took me about 3 years to return to my pre–pregnancy weight, but in those three years, everything about how I view diet, movement, supplementation, and our food culture changed.

I grew up eating a typical standard American diet (SAD). We always had protein, starch and vegetables on our plates. We cooked burgers, ate omelets, and drank beer. My parents did instill some good food values which I continue to this day, including moderation of sweets and emphasis on protein. But it also instilled a lot of anxiety on me as I entered into parenthood.

Growing up in the U.S., being inundated with food marketing campaigns, fad diets, and the almighty FDA food pyramid, and then spending a decade dedicated to counting protein and macros, it was incredibly difficult to shift my perspective. Even today, as I'm writing this in my fourth year of parenthood, I still have anxiety around what my kids are eating.

We are getting used to the idea that raw fruits and veggies are a nutritious and appropriate meal, and we don't try to force the SAD plate design in our home anymore.

Throughout my military career, my diet went from the typical SAD to a spectrum of variations of Paleo, Carnivore, Keto, and the typical bodybuilding diet of rice, potatoes, lean meat and cruciferous veggies (weighed and measured, of course).

In 2020, when I was exiting the military, I would have told you I was very healthy, and I believed it. I also smoked cigarettes and drank liberal amounts of alcohol during most of my career, with alcohol being a significant coping mechanism for me during the heights of my trauma symptoms. I was also incredibly strong, attractive, and didn't have any health issues aside from my mental health struggles, so anyone else would tell you I was healthy as well.

In 2022, I discovered psychedelic medicine, and for the first time in more than a decade, started to feel genuine relief from my mental health symptoms. Like most things I do, I dove in head first, learning everything I could about psilocybin mushrooms, how they're cultivated, how they work in the brain and body, and how to integrate with them.

My diet improved by association, and I began to relieve myself of all pharmaceutical medicines as well, learning about plant medicine on a wider level and realizing much of what I needed in my home pharmacopeia lives all around me. I started losing weight without trying, despite abstaining from counting calories… eating intuitively as I cared for my babies.

As I progressed through my self–treatment, things started to line up, but it also required me to reconsider everything I believed to be true about my world and how it functioned.

Toward the end of 2023, I turned to a plant-based diet to see what I may benefit from it. Plant-based is all the rage these days, with the Impossible Burger, and honestly, a vast improvement in packaged food options for individuals with dietary sensitivities… but my goal was to be as whole food, raw, plant based as possible, and stick to local options.

I described myself as a militant atheist for most of my life, but after a few larger doses of psilocybin, I could not unsee the reality of what exists beneath the surface of consciousness, and my partner and I began an intensely loving spiritual journey, guided by intuition and plant medicine. Deciding to go plant–based was less about what I was going to eat, and more about what I was going to remove as far as low vibration energy.

On the fall solstice of 2023, I quit consumption of meat, dairy, and alcohol cold turkey. During that year, I lost about 35 pounds, finally achieving my pre–pregnancy weight. Most of the weight loss came after shifting my diet, and the change in my body was astounding.

I was significantly smaller, fitting into clothes from before I was pregnant, but weighed the same. I had assumed it was because my body composition was different now. But the way people reacted to my weight loss was telling. Most people who mentioned it said they noticed it because they saw it in my hands or my face.

I realized I had lost weight too fast for it to have been body fat. I had an epiphany that had always been under the surface with my education in fitness and health – I hadn't really been "fat" this whole time; I had been suffering from inflammation.

I looked back at pictures of myself from the last decade and was surprised by how "puffy" I looked. My perspective on my past body changed, as well as my perspective on my new body. I wasn't that healthy; I was barely functioning through a massive, chronic inflammatory response from what I was putting in my body and what I was being exposed to in the military.

Something incredibly surprising happened during this dietary shift as well. Almost all of my mental health symptoms disappeared. Prior to that solstice, I was regularly suffering from PTSD symptoms, including debilitating suicidal ideation. These episodes reduced significantly after finding plant medicine, but they still plagued me and my family on a regular basis. Removing alcohol, meat and dairy sent my condition into remission, and for the first time in my life I felt truly like myself. It felt as though I were meeting myself for the first time, and I was able to see that so much of who I am is written in pencil, not pen.

I still struggled with the neurodivergence of PTSD (or maybe ADHD), but it became easier for me to be honest about what I needed and what "style" of human I am. I struggled with providing a healthy, wholesome diet to my family, but realized I need to cultivate the same intuitive connection to self in my kids. What can I impart onto them that will stick with them long term and help them navigate a world full of toxic enticement? I don't have the answer; I'm writing the answer as I go.

How do I know these three foods were essentially the "cause" of my symptoms? Obviously, I don't. But, I do have a few tells. Obviously, alcohol is a toxic drug that was very likely contributing to my symptoms, and my abstinence is important to me. Alcohol is one of those substances that doesn't produce satiety – the more you drink, the more you want to drink. We all understand that, but it felt different in my body at this point. I started to apply that reasoning to everything else I consumed.

The food we eat should make us feel good, and we shouldn't want to overindulge on it. Food that aligns in our body should have a healthy limit to it, eating it shouldn't entice us to eat more and more of it. I realized I had this same reaction when eating wheat–based foods, as well as with dairy and sugar.

My relationship with meat and dairy also shifted from a spiritual perspective. My journey with plant medicine showed me that my relationship with these foods was not serving me. Dairy, especially, operated the same as alcohol in my body – the more I eat it, the more I want it. Dairy, I also discovered, was a catalyst for my PTSD symptoms. In the spring of 2024, I had an accidental exposure to dairy after eating food I thought was dairy-free, but wasn't. A few days later, I was inundated with anxiety and flashbacks, something I hadn't experienced in several months. I abstained from dairy again and my symptoms subsided.

It may be the hormone profile of dairy products or maybe the quality of the dairy I was eating. It could have been the quantity or the source. The only thing I really miss about eating dairy is the convenience, so I'm not interested in finding out the true mechanism of this association. I learned an old, possibly Hindu belief that resonated with me on a spiritual level, "dairy is the energy of rape." The dairy industry is rife with unethical practices, impregnating cattle and extending their lactation process through artificial means to procure the most profitable outcomes. From this perspective, I would not benefit from associating with practices that cause this type of harm.

Also in the spring of 2024, plant medicine encouraged me to try meat again. I have Ehlers Danlos Syndrome, and started feeling like I was struggling nutritionally. My connective tissue disorder can't be treated supplementally, but I had a feeling that I would fare better with some animal protein. Since then, I've incorporated some local, ethically sourced red meat into my diet a few times a month, along with local eggs. I try to maintain a whole food, plant based diet as my staples, with thoughtful supplementation of foods that align with my values.

Short term abstinence is one of the most significant practices I've developed during my healing journey. If my partner and I start to get a sense that something we're doing is bordering on dysfunctional, we have no issue abstaining from it for a while. This can include activities, the use of substances like cannabis, over–the–counter medications (which we still use when necessary), or food.

We also aim to source our food as locally as possible, especially fermented foods, of which a few I have started to master, like kombucha, sourdough, and fire cider.

I recently did a gluten fast for six weeks just to see how it might affect my body. It was a good opportunity for me to practice this idea of abstinence in real time, and while I still consume gluten foods, it did help to teach me more about food, where it comes from, and how it works. It was through this abstinence period that I understood my association with wheat foods and disruption in satiety, as my desire to overindulge on chickpea pasta was not present like it was with wheat-based pasta and other foods.

Something I tell those who I mentor through diet, movement or plant medicine, is that if its presence or its absence feels distressing to you, there's something there to explore.

Many people I speak to have an automatic reaction when I tell them I don't eat dairy. First, they assume I have some type of intolerance or allergy to it. Then, they tell me that they do have an intolerance to dairy, but they eat it anyway, even though it makes them feel awful, or forces them to take medicine to manage it.

The emotional attachment to dairy, meat, and sugar in our country makes me concerned, especially after noticing how my mental health improved without it.

Ultimately, my healing journey is based largely on cultivating relationships. These relationships are with people, animals, environments, food, supplements, activities, and habits. I take the time to ask myself "what am I putting into my body, and why?" This could be food, media, information, time, or energy. It's understanding that more of something doesn't equal better.

As we can have toxic relationships with people; we can develop a toxic relationship with anything else we encounter in our lives. Our relationships with everything around us reflects our own self-worth. To be relational with our habits and inputs is to create a living document, a contract that offers respect, care, and thought for our health and well-being.

We know how the story ends, and we are writing it as we go.

EDITOR'S NOTES: KEY TAKEAWAYS FROM KALI'S STORY

- We can get so enmeshed in diet plans that we lose sight of the forest because we're so busy counting the trees. Accountability to health plans is important, but we do not need to be weighing ourselves or our daily calorie intake, nor keeping a spreadsheet of all the macronutrients we consume.
- Many people can appear healthy on the outside in terms of appearance, while inside systems are failing, leading to chronic inflammation and a host of other deadly illnesses. Being overweight or obese is an outward sign of ill health, but looks alone are insufficient.

- Changing to a healthy diet and lifestyle can lead to no longer needing pharmaceutical drugs that are simply helping you manage problematic symptoms; once you heal the underlying problems, the symptoms "magically" disappear and drugs are no longer necessary. (But always consult with your doctor before stopping any prescription drugs.)
- Diet flexibility is a hallmark of the Healing Revolution Diet! The goal is to only eat foods that support your health – the health of your body, gut, and brain – but those foods need to be regularly analyzed and evaluated, especially when things change or you start feeling differently (truly a gut intuition) about certain foods.

CHAPTER FIFTEEN
Chris' Story

MOVING TO A HIGHER VIBRATION!

Name: Chris Peskuski

How do you feel (mentally and physically) now? I am sturdier and more resilient than ever. Happier, healthier, and stronger than I've ever been, hands down. I'm more present and clearer-headed than ever in my life.

How were you (mentally and physically) before you started? Completely demoralized very depressed. Fat, unkept, uncaring, distracted, self-medicating. I'd become a victim and I was spiraling downhill quickly. I spent a lot of time worrying about the future and reliving the past – and wasn't paying much attention to the present. I held a ton of shame, regret, guilt, fear, and stress.

Best aspect of your plan: Keeping an open mind and learning! Not getting locked into any single modality. Being willing to change consistently. When things aren't working anymore, change it up! My wife describes me as a student. I have some healthy role models and always challenge what I know in all aspects of life.

Hardest part of your plan: Setbacks. I've had a few back and knee injuries. Being sensitive to what I need. Cooking and eating slowly because convenience kills.

Key indicators of your health and healing: My relationships are much better. Mental clarity and presence, general attitude and outlook on life, blood pressure, strength, mobility, and weight loss!

Biggest surprise of your health journey: How everything is connected and how important it is to live an examined life and to be spiritually well. Having a philosophy matters. How we've become a victim to convenience and circumstance because it's easy, but also because we've been conditioned to be so.

If we want to change the world around us, we must first change ourselves.

I grew up in the East Mountains of Albuquerque, New Mexico, in a household where there was a lot of love from my parents. They're great, wonderful people who were doing the best they could, dealing with their own issues and childhood trauma.

That said, there were a lot of drugs and alcohol in my house too. My parents were young and often intoxicated – and weren't paying as much attention to me as they probably should have been. (Along my healing journey I've come to realize how much both of my parents are dealing with intergenerational traumas).

There was always food on the table, though it wasn't always the highest quality and it was mostly processed foods. It was especially bad when my mom was going to school as my dad wasn't a good cook back then. We ate a lot of mac and cheese during those times. But, at least we mostly ate at home. When we did eat out, it was the cheap burritos from Taco Bell. If we went to a restaurant, it was usually Mexican food… beans, tortillas, cheese. I wouldn't say any of it was high quality stuff.

That's the kind of diet I had growing up. Lots of pasta and occasionally some healthy foods. My parents tried to grow a garden a couple of times. By high school, the food at home got a little better with more vegetables – but mostly canned, not fresh.

I had a lot of aggressive urges as a kid and no good outlets for dealing with it, and my parents didn't know how to handle it very well. They did get me into martial arts once. But with them struggling with their own issues, it wasn't a priority and it was actually discouraged in a lot of ways because it was inconvenient and a pain in the butt to get me to classes.

After high school, I lived on my own for a bit, working and living in a little trailer at the job site. I had started drinking in high school, and now the drinking ramped up. I was eating absolute crap foods, like stovetop stuffing and the like.

During that time, I was not addressing my aggressive energy very well, and it was manifesting itself in bad, self-destructive ways. So around 2003, I decided I had to do something drastic or else I was going to end up in prison. That's what led me to join the Marines, where they seemed to appreciate that aggressive energy; it was welcomed and channeled in a healthier way.

In the Marine Corps, I was still eating unhealthily. I mean, even when they were trying to upgrade some of their food facilities, it was still Sodexo – a traditional food services company and not that high quality. Thus, the diet I was eating while in the Marines was Sodexo and fast food.

I got married while in the Marines and my wife was the first person who brought organic food to my attention. But at the time my attitude was that we can't feed 8 billion people with organic food. We need all the conventional foods. I now realize I was simply buying into the lies, drinking the Kool-Aid. That was around 2006 when she started introducing that into my life, and we were both fairly healthy for a little while because of her influence.

Unfortunately, my drinking was getting a lot worse – especially after I'd gotten back from Iraq, where I'd been blown up multiple times. My job in the Marines was a forward observer, so I was responsible for calling in artillery attacks and airstrikes. We lost some people in my unit. The deaths and injuries I witnessed along with general war trauma compounded my drinking problem, and compromised my mental health.

I was struggling with doing my job, but I was hesitant to admit any of these weaknesses to myself – or anybody else. I was masking it all with alcohol and becoming more scared all the time. It took a toll on me.

I then served in Afghanistan, and got blown up there. I was losing it. Unfortunately, the Marine Corps doesn't care. They're chewing people up as fast as they can. It's all about mission accomplishment.

After I got out of Afghanistan, I decided to leave the Marines. I was scaring the shit out of myself doing what I was doing and barely holding on. That was in 2011.

I had trouble with my transition into the civilian world. I was disillusioned with everything.

At least in the Marines, there was some structure that was channeling a lot of my aggressive energy in a useful way. I had camaraderie and structure, which was holding me together. But then I got out and came into the civilian world. I started to become demoralized, wondering what it was I had been fighting for. It felt like a fricking train wreck, but I was emotionally numb to my own stuff. You just have to do what you do to survive.

I felt like I was going into some deep depression, so I started self-medicating with other things aside from alcohol… just trying to hold my shit together. To help me with focus, I got a prescription for Adderall and Modafinil and I was self-medicating with Tramadol and alcohol at night.

I had lots of highs and lows, ups and downs, but overall, going downhill fast. Well, I guess not fast. It took a decade. It was a long decade of highs and lows. My wife tried to intervene and help me get out of the depression, but it was not much help.

I kept searching for solutions. I finally found EMDR therapy that helped a little bit.

Meanwhile, our eating habits were up and down, but mostly the traditional American diet: eating some fast food and eating conveniently and conventionally. I gained a lot of weight and was struggling with heartburn issues and drinking a lot of diet sodas. Interestingly, any type of artificial sweetener gives me bad heartburn now.

Then Covid hit and I started working from home, and I would get my snack on all day, working right next to the fridge. Not only eating all day, but also eating a lot of prepacked, processed foods… just eating mindlessly while working.

With both my wife and I working from home at the same time, it led me to drinking a lot more – and it was all bad. But then there was a good stretch of time where I was traveling a lot for work; I was gone every other week for six months. During that time, I was eating gas station food. I can chuckle about it now because even my young son knows better. Just after Covid, when he was with me, I decided to grab some food from the gas station store and he told me he thought the idea of getting food from a gas station was silly. And he's right.

Sadly, while traveling for work, I did eat a lot of gas station food – and had gotten to about 270 pounds.

But I didn't care. That was the biggest thing. I didn't care about myself anymore. In some ways, I think I was feeling all the guilt and shit from being an alcoholic for most of my life. And, I think, for some of the stuff that happened in Iraq and Afghanistan, I was probably trying to punish myself.

Finally, I remember taking a good hard look at myself in the mirror and thinking, how the hell did I get here? But then, because I was feeding myself a yummy diet of Modafinil and Adderall, I would work for a whole week without eating much, and accidentally lost weight.

So, during those 10 years or so, my weight fluctuated up and down.

I knew I needed more help. I thought about Transcranial Magnetic Stimulation (TMS), but all the research I did on that kind of scared me. I had used psychedelics a little bit from time to time, and even though I wasn't using it in an intentional way, it still seemed to help me.

It was then that ayahuasca started calling to me.

I wanted to go through Heroic Hearts Project (HHP) for healing, but at the time their waitlist was too long… and I could not wait. I decided to go to the Arkana Spiritual Center based on one of HHP's videos. I ended up finding my way down there last November.

I did six ayahuasca ceremonies, and shattered myself in one of them. The medicine picked me apart piece by piece and showed me that I was being a victim in a lot of ways, but that I was a warrior at heart, and that I've been weak and I needed to get my shit together because I got work to do. Awesome.

I'm still not sure what my life's work is, but I've been working on myself ever since in every way. I now feel so fantastic. Fantastic!

Before attending the ayahuasca retreat, my blood pressure was through the roof. My weight was my heaviest and I was wheezing just bending over to tie my shoes. I remember trying to get my blood pressure down before going to my retreat. I was going to acupuncture, anything I could do to get my blood pressure down, but in the end, I decided that I had to just go there. I thought to myself, if I die down there, so be it, but I'm going to fricking die here if I don't get my shit together.

I knew I had to do something because everything was going downhill at that point.

With ayahuasca, participants are supposed to follow a "dieta" of extremely healthy and clean eating – and that was the beginning of food change for me. The dieta gave me a chance to have a good hard look at everything I was eating and I decided to continue a bunch of the tenets of the dieta after returning home. For example, I haven't eaten any beef or pork since my retreat.

I did try to go vegetarian for a little while, but it wasn't working for me. I wasn't getting enough protein. Now that I know a bit more about plant-based proteins, I might try again, but my focus is on eating high-quality food, organic food everywhere I can – and shopping more locally at the farmer's market.

We're now a family that prioritizes health and wellness. My wife has been trying for years to do that, but I was not on board. I was lying on the couch depressed and/or out being a drunken fool somewhere.

And while the food is a big component, it's just one of several. One of my best wellness practices is meditation; it's teaching me how to master my mind – and that's just as important as mastering my body. The body and mind must both be healed.

Today, I'm stronger and healthier physically than I've been in a long time. Spiritually, philosophically, and emotionally, I'm way better than I've ever been.

I still have work to do in all aspects of life, particularly physically and emotionally. I'm working on it every day. I try to live an examined life from a place of love and joy and be the change I want to see in the world.

I do at least three things for myself every day! Some of my practices include: meditation, working out, breathing, martial arts, cold and heat exposure, walking, art, sound baths, Reiki treatments, getting time in the sunshine, reading a book about something inspirational, listening to binaural beats, acupuncture treatment, developing relationships, doing community service, gift giving, doing a fast or giving something up, doing something hard or scary, going to therapy.

All of these things help move me either physically, emotionally, mentally, or spiritually and movement is the key to living in higher vibration.

I truly believe that we can change the world by changing ourselves.

EDITOR'S NOTES: KEY TAKEAWAYS FROM CHRIS' STORY

- Convenience is literally a killer, especially with food. People typically eat the worst foods (such as "gas station foods") when we are under time pressure and/or on the road. These imposter foods found in all food stores and fast food restaurants are only good for packing on the pounds and building toxins in your body that can lead to serious health conditions and a slow death.

- With education and/or the help of a supportive partner, we can overcome a lack of knowledge from our childhood about food, cooking, nutrition. It takes work and support from all family members, as well as some trial-and-error, but the journey to health and real foods is worth it.

- Trauma plays a serious role in poor habits, including self-medicating with drugs and alcohol, which is why healing past trauma wounds is essential. With food, whether consciously or not, we often feel we need and deserve ultra-processed "comfort foods" even when we know how bad they are for us; or it can work the other way: that we're so broken that what's the point in "wasting" money on quality foods.

- So many of us have been brainwashed into thinking that conventional farming is "saving the world," but the world does not need the massive amounts of corn, soybean, and wheat monocrops nor the small amount of conventionally-grown fruits and vegetables. Conventional farming destroys the soil, coats the crops in chemical fertilizers, pesticides, and herbicides, and contributes to erosion and water runoff. Regenerative organic farming will save and feed the world – and do it in a way that replenishes the soil, making the foods raised all the more nutrient-dense.

CHAPTER SIXTEEN
Mandy's Story

NEVER LOOKING BACK

Name: Mandy Rodrigues

How do you feel (mentally and physically) now? Great! Mentally very clear, no more fog! Physically very good; I feel stronger and healthier at 44 than I did at 34.

How were you (mentally and physically) before you started? In bad shape. One doctor even told me I was a ticking time bomb physically. Mentally, I was foggy, moody, and unhappy.

Best aspect of your plan: No counting or tracking calories or macros, unlimited fruits and veggies, and what's good for me is also good for the environment.

Hardest part of your plan: Dealing with others' judgment of my food choices.

Key indicators of your health and healing: My quality of sleep has greatly improved, my mental clarity is sharp, and my yearly bloodwork now serves as a reliable baseline for my health.

Biggest surprise of your health journey: How simple it was once I educated myself and followed the science. I've realized that I can control my weight simply through food choices.

I feel so lucky when I reflect on my childhood. We were a blue-collar family in New Jersey; my mom was an elementary school teacher and my dad worked in the family business (a local bar/grill) that his parents opened in 1945.

We weren't rich by any means, but we always had food on the table, took summer vacations, and our parents worked very hard to give us everything they could.

It was the late 1980s, and by the third grade, I loved everything about sports and physical activity. Before I reached middle school, I was playing girls' softball, little league baseball, co-ed soccer, volleyball, basketball, and I was even in a bowling league.

At one point, my younger brother and I were on the same little league baseball team. I was competitive and loved to be outside, moving! No matter how busy we were, my parents always made sure we had family meals around the table.

In my opinion, the meals were pretty healthy and always "hit the food groups." There was always some type of protein like a piece of chicken or a pork chop, a grain (typically mashed potatoes), and a veggie. I remember string beans, broccoli, or peas and carrots being regulars on my plate.

My mother made great homemade tomato sauce and meatballs, which were fantastic with our pasta, sometimes accompanied by bread and butter. Friday nights were our takeout nights, usually pizza or Chinese food delivery, so my parents could relax after working all week.

Fast forward to the mid-1990s, and I was a high school varsity athlete playing volleyball and softball in programs that were highly competitive and winning state championships. My nightly dinners were still pretty good, but school lunch consisted of grilled cheese, chicken fingers and fries, sub sandwiches… and I was a Coca-Cola addict.

Despite this, I took pride in never falling into peer pressure with smoking or drinking. I had many high school friends who smoked and drank, but I never got involved in that. I always remember thinking, "That's not good for you."

This trend continued into college. I was recruited to play NCAA volleyball, and throughout my collegiate career, even in the off-season, I never tried tobacco, pot, or had a sip of alcohol. I was the designated driver for everyone, which made me very popular with my teammates, but I also consciously felt good about being a college athlete and not doing anything that could hinder my performance.

In 2002, after graduating from college, I started my career as a physical education and health teacher. I loved teaching health to my students, especially the cardiovascular system and how important our heart is. I would create all kinds of projects to get them as excited as I was to learn about their bodies and prioritize their personal health.

Of course, I coached sports after school, and I even continued playing competitive volleyball in a women's league filled with many former college athletes. I always prided myself on setting the example of being active until…

Ten years later, with 20 varsity coaching seasons behind me, I decided to go all in and open a business with my coaching partner. We opened a competitive travel volleyball program for athletes, which involved traveling all over the country.

This was in addition to maintaining my teaching job.

So, let me paint the picture for you: Up at 6:30 a.m., commute to work and teach from 8 a.m. to 3 p.m., commute back home, grab a snack, and then run the business from 4 p.m. to 10:30 p.m.

Dinner… hmm… whatever was open at 10:30 p.m. – usually pizza, Chinese, or whatever fast food had a drive-thru. I would slam it down and watch TV from 11:00 p.m. to midnight. Sleep from midnight to 6:30 a.m., and hit the repeat button.

Weekends were no better, and 1-2 times a month I was flying with our travel volleyball teams to tournaments across the country – from Atlanta, Georgia, to Denver, Colorado; Dallas, Texas; Indianapolis, Indiana, and more.

Imagine the airport food and on-the-road food options… not the greatest. Sleep deprivation was an understatement. This went on for an entire year, and as year two of our business started, we had doubled our athletes and teams, which meant more weekend hours, more flights to tournaments, less sleep, and more airport cuisine. EEK!

During this second year, I started noticing I was living on coffee and Advil during the day at my teaching job. My lack of sleep and diet packed with simple carbs and sugar had me crashing and burning, leading to daily headaches.

I was becoming a less-than-acceptable teacher and definitely not modeling what I was teaching in my health classes. I also started to get into the mindset of being proud to be a workaholic, like it was a badge of honor.

As the end of our second year approached, my business partner and I started looking for a new facility to support the capacity we knew was coming in year three. Our 4,000 square feet of gym space was bursting at the seams, and we were looking at places of 12,000-15,000 square feet to start a new lease and continue to grow our business. We were excited about what we had built, and again, we were proud to be "hard workers."

Teaching full-time and owning/running a business was *how we were going to be successful*.

By the spring of 2014, I realized I had spiraled out of control. I don't remember the exact day, but I remember realizing my entire wardrobe consisted of bulky sweatpants and sweatshirts because none of my other clothes fit anymore. I weighed myself, and I was *disgusted*. At 5'7", I had ballooned up to over 230 pounds. I also noticed I was frequently winded and felt completely exhausted.

Advil was now a side dish to my coffee and fast food. At one point, I was taking 6-8 Advil daily for the headaches. One day at work, I felt horrible. I looked in the mirror and realized my neck was completely broken out in hives. I went to the school nurse, and she took my blood pressure, which was through the roof. She recommended I see a doctor ASAP, but of course, I had no time for that because I had to work.

I continued my normal schedule: up early, teaching job, drive home, run the business, fast food, repeat.

One day, I got home from teaching, grabbed a quick snack before leaving for volleyball practice at my business, when all of a sudden, I had the worst headache I'd ever experienced. It came out of nowhere –

the room started to spin, and the pain intensified until it seemed to culminate in what I can only describe as a burst, and then I passed out. I don't think I was out for long, maybe a minute or two, but when I came to, the headache worsened. I probably should have gone to a hospital, but instead, I laid down, took a handful of Advil, and eventually the pain subsided.

I made a doctor's appointment the next day.

At 34 years old, I was a health and physical education teacher – a former collegiate athlete who prided herself on health – yet I was now sitting in my follow-up appointment getting my lab results. I was still more than 230 pounds – and was now being told I had severe high blood pressure, was pre-diabetic, had a total cholesterol near 250, and triglycerides above 300.

The doctor said I was insane not to have gone to a hospital after my episode because, based on what I described, she said I could have had a stroke or a severe thunderclap headache, which could have caused bleeding in my brain.

She told me I was going to need a prescription for my blood pressure and strongly advised cutting back on work. In her words, "You are what we call a widow maker in progress."

This was my rock bottom, my moment of realization: "I'm done. I can't live to work, or I will work myself to death."

I refused the prescription and told her I would take care of it and come back in six months. She strongly advised against it, but I promised that if I didn't improve in six months, I would take the medication.

I started reading everything I could find about cardiovascular health, diabetes, and lifestyle changes. I explored weight loss without medication, holistic approaches to healing the body, and ways to exercise without needing a gym membership.

The Mediterranean Diet kept coming up in my search as a popular and effective way to get healthy. I found countless articles explaining how unlimited fruits and vegetables could not only reverse aspects of heart disease but also prevent weight gain due to their high fiber content and low-calorie density.

I began making and eating loaded salads with kale, spinach, and a variety of veggies like broccoli, peppers, and carrots, along with nuts and seeds such as pumpkin seeds and chia seeds. I'd even toss in some chopped apples and almonds.

These meals made me feel full but not stuffed. Inspired to learn more, I signed up for a certificate program at Cornell on plant-based nutrition and its impact on reversing chronic disease. That course was my turning point – the moment I knew I would never look back. The information was eye-opening, and the science made perfect sense to me.

From that point on, I removed all meat, eggs, and dairy milk from my diet. Fast food became a thing of the past. While I still occasionally ate fish and cheese, my diet primarily consisted of fruits, veggies, nuts, and seeds.

I also started walking daily for exercise, and after a couple of months, I was covering a couple of miles a day. After about three months, I fully committed and stopped eating fish and cheese altogether. I stuck to what I had learned at Cornell, and I continued educating myself by reading numerous articles and books. The weight began to fall off, my mental clarity improved, and I was excited to return to the doctor for my six-month check-up.

When my doctor entered the room, she immediately asked, "What are you doing?" I told her about my plant-based nutrition courses and how I had read the science and embraced it. She was floored – my weight had dropped from more than 230 pounds down to 175 in just six months.

Then she reviewed my lab results. WOW, I couldn't believe it! My total cholesterol was down to the 160s, triglycerides under 200, and my A1C was 4.7 – practically off the chart in a good way, nowhere near pre-diabetic. She admitted she didn't think I would return and had expected me to become a statistic.

It's now ten years later, and I've never looked back. I've been plant-based ever since.

People often ask if I've gained weight back because they don't believe that eating plant-based is sustainable. My weight has fluctuated by about 10 pounds up and down, but it's always due to the same issue: eating frozen vegan foods out of convenience. As soon as I return to eating whole plant foods, the weight melts right off again.

This is important for people to understand – *vegan doesn't automatically mean healthy* – which is why I always focus on eating a whole food plant-based diet.

Mandy Rodrigues is a private consultant who works with individuals and organizations on change and wellness, an ongoing student of health and medicine, and a former university professor of health and human performance, who supports those looking for strategies and scientifically proven ways to improve their health. Find Mandy on LinkedIn: https://www.linkedin.com/in/mandy-rodrigues/

EDITOR'S NOTES: KEY TAKEAWAYS FROM MANDY'S STORY

- Being/staying active can help disguise poor eating and a sugar addiction, which can actually lead to a more dangerous health situation once the activity slows or stops. No one can exercise their way out of a bad diet.
- Even someone educated in health can be overwhelmed by life's obligations and the related stress, especially chronic stress.
- Poor diet, especially one filled with simple carbohydrates and sugar, can wreak havoc on the body – and brain.
- It's never too late to attempt to reverse chronic health conditions (such as high blood pressure, excess weight, pre-diabetic, diabetes type 2) with proper nutrition, diet, and lifestyle.

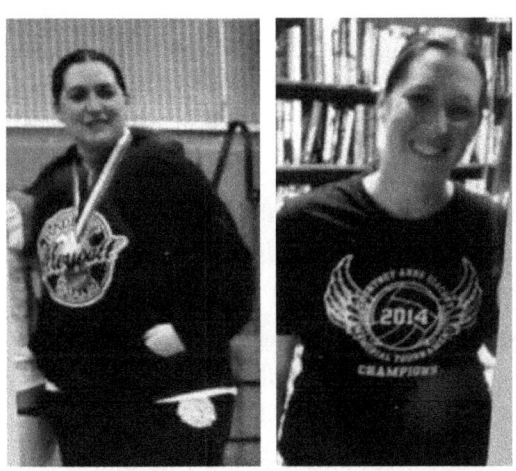

(left) Spring 2014-approx 1-2 months before I passed out with the severe pain in my head.
(right) Summer 2015, what a difference a year makes!

CHAPTER SEVENTEEN

Emily's Story

HEALING AFTER 20+ YEARS OF FAILED MENTAL HEALTH TREATMENTS

Name: Emily Anne Herrick

How do you feel (mentally and physically) now? Better than I did when I was 20 years old – both mentally and physically. My worst days now are far better than any of the days I used to have.

How were you (mentally and physically) before you started? My life was a wreck. I had severe treatment-resistant depression, my anxiety was overwhelming, I had uncontrolled asthma, and I was obese. Today, I don't deal with any of these things; for the past 8 years, I've experienced freedom I didn't know was possible.

Best aspect of your plan: The food I eat tastes great, is satisfying, and I'm never hungry. It's also a simple way to eat! I like simple; it gives me more time to be outdoors or spend time with my family.

Hardest part of your plan: Social gatherings. So much of how we celebrate and interact in society revolves around food. I have to make sure I plan carefully and set good boundaries around what I can and can't eat.

Key indicators of your health and healing: I no longer take any medications or have the need for a team of medical professionals. I see one integrative doctor who monitors my lab work and helps keep my hormones balanced, but otherwise I have put all my chronic medical and former mental health conditions into remission. With the exception of my hormones (which fluctuate due to perimenopause), all my labs are normal.

Biggest surprise of your health journey: How wrong medical advice is regarding the underlying causes of so many mental and physical health symptoms. And how disinterested they are in learning – even my former doctors who know I got better just aren't interested in knowing HOW it happened.

I want to start my story by sharing that I grew up in a middle-class family, probably upper middle class. Once I started experiencing issues, my parents were always willing to send me to whatever therapist or doctor for help. I think that's one of the things about my story that's unique. I really did have what was considered the best help available, and it still wasn't enough to help me.

My mental health struggles started when I was really young. I remember being seven years old and lying in bed at night and having chest pains and thinking, oh gosh, am I going to die? Not knowing what was going on, my mom took me to the doctor. They said I was fine. It wasn't until many, many years later that I realized that what I was experiencing was anxiety, that I was having panic attacks at a very young age.

When it comes to nutrition while growing up, I think the quality of everything that we had to eat in the 1980s was probably considerably better than it has been the last decade or two. That said, I grew up where dinner might be a grilled cheese sandwich, chips for snacks. We probably did McDonald's and Taco Bell a couple of times a week.

When I was younger, I didn't eat a lot of vegetables or fruits, but physically I felt okay. I was very active, athletic, and didn't have any physical health problems in terms of being overweight or obese. I had good energy, but the anxiety was always there.

By the age of 12, I started to experience low mood. I didn't call it depression, but that's definitely what it was. So by the age of 12 or 13, I had both anxiety *and* depression. I never want to discount that there were some difficult things in my childhood happening beyond my control that influenced all of this.

Without getting into the specifics, there were some traumatic things in my childhood. Still, the amount of anxiety that I always seemed to carry felt a lot bigger than was warranted, given the circumstances I was going through.

So, by age 13, I was put on an antidepressant. Unfortunately, things got worse. My moods became more erratic. I developed an eating disorder, bulimia, which involved consuming tons and tons of processed foods on a daily basis.

Thus, my teenage years were filled with anxiety, depression, mood swings, *and* an eating disorder.

I went to college and things started to get worse. I was taking trips to treatment facilities for eating disorders or being hospitalized for my severe depression, along with some suicidal ideation. I never wanted to kill myself, but I did have suicidal thoughts. But these thoughts scared me because I wanted to live.

I always wanted to get better; I had this strong desire to get better.

I shuffled between different antidepressants. Eventually benzodiazepines were added. I quickly built up a high tolerance to them, had to detox off of them, and started taking other psychiatric medications – just different combinations of drugs.

My twenties were decent; some years were okay, but none were good. I graduated from college, though it took me six years. I also worked as a social worker at this time.

In my late twenties, I got married. I had this odd experience right afterward where I developed debilitating joint pain and fatigue; it was so bad I couldn't get out of bed without a lot of effort. I went to my doctors, and they gave me some sort of arthritis diagnosis, a lifelong condition. The doctors gave me a prescription for medications, but they didn't help.

I was still struggling with my eating disorder and at some point, I realized I was drinking about a case of diet Dr. Pepper a day. I recognized that it might be the aspartame in the diet soda, so I cut it off and switched the soda out for plain fizzy water. All of that joint pain went away fairly quicky, and that was my first kind of "aha" moment of what I'm putting in my body can really affect how I feel.

But that connection didn't translate over into all these other areas of my life until a bit later.

In my early thirties, I got pregnant and had a son. Shortly after he was born, things got really, really bad. I had severe postpartum depression.

My mental health was actually a little bit better while I was pregnant, probably because I was on a lot less medication. I don't think my food changed a lot then.

After the birth, I also had insulin resistance and was pre-diabetic. My weight had risen to about 240 pounds.

With my postpartum depression, it is a miracle I survived, but luckily I found this holistic psychiatrist. I had once again been put on several medications and she asked whether anyone had tested my hormone levels. (The answer was no.) She recommended I get tested by my regular doctor, who prescribed progesterone. That bioidentical progesterone was instrumental; it was key to helping pull me out of that depression.

But for my other issues, I ended up going right back to the people and places I had been before. Same professionals, same facilities. I went to all these places and nobody could help me.

Then one night it all came to an end.

I ended up in the emergency room with severe chest pains.

The ER doctor asked me why I was on all these medications. That question was like an awakening for me. I didn't know what to tell him, but to myself, I thought, "why am I on all these medications and what if there's another way?"

That night I turned to the internet to see if there were any alternatives. I was searching for anyone doing something different who could finally help me.

During this time, I had gotten a master's degree in social work, so I knew the limitations of what the conventional system had to offer. I'm not against therapy. There's a time and place for it, but if therapy was going to be my answer, I would've worked that out already.

So I ended up finding this group of online professionals and they started telling me about food. They suggested that my diet could be playing a role, and recommended I start something like a *Whole 30* diet, which I did. In the beginning I really struggled, but I did notice as I started coming off my prescribed medications and as I changed my diet, I began to feel *a whole lot better*.

I realized through this process of trying different foods that gluten was the biggest trigger for my depression and the anxiety. Even with that knowledge, it took me several starts and stops before I stuck to a gluten-free diet.

I had this moment of clarity where I realized I would have to go back on medication that wasn't working, but was keeping my anxiety from totally spinning out of control, or I would to have to decide that being gluten-free was my new way of life.

When I realized that, I quit gluten. It's been eight years since I've had any gluten. And I have not needed a hospital. I have not needed a psychiatrist. I have not taken a psychiatric med. I have been able to completely control all of my mental health symptoms through diet alone. I also had been on medication for a form of thyroiditis that I no longer needed once I eliminated gluten from my diet.

Everything was good, except for occasional intrusive thoughts that hung with me. I didn't know where those came from, but happily I found the work of Dr. Christopher Palmer. (Dr. Palmer is a pioneer in the use of the ketogenic diet and its applications in psychiatry.)

I was amazed because a ketogenic diet, within a couple of weeks to a month, reduced those intrusive thoughts.

I had high hopes of it working because I had already tried so many medications and knew they weren't the answer.

Thus, for the past couple of years, I've been following a low-carb, ketogenic diet. And for the past eight years, my depression and my anxiety have been well controlled. My asthma disappeared as well, and I have had no further issues with bulimia.

I have changed my relationship with food to where I see food as food is medicine. That sounds kind of cliche, right?

I don't know that food is medicine. *It's more than medicine.*

Food is the message that I give my body for how I want to feel and think – everything about me physically, emotionally, and mentally is determined based on how I'm eating.

So yes, I have changed my relationship with food because it is the most important decision I make on a daily basis. What am I going to eat today? The answer is critical because it's that important to how well I function and feel.

The importance of diet is something that people don't realize, especially in the mental health world. Hopefully that's changing, but there *are* people like me who are very sensitive to all of these things. Diet can and does have a major impact. Another example is that I can't use stevia instead of sugar because for whatever reasons, I become extremely irritable for long periods after consuming it.

Everybody has to try out what foods work best for their bodies and brains. I try to be really careful when I am sharing my story that I'm not coming off as stating that there is one diet that everybody must use because I don't believe that.

People have to find the kinds of foods that work for them, for their health. And I think that those can change over time.

I don't know if I will do keto forever. I do know that I will be gluten-free forever if I want to have any measure of mental well-being. But for the rest, I don't know. *I plan to take it as it comes.*

What I can say is all my labs are great since being gluten-free and on the keto diet. Everything's improved.

I practically live off a diet of meat and eggs and fat, and it's just so amazing what being in ketosis does for the brain and the body.

I emphasize with others who are struggling. It can be really hard because a lot of these medications I took made me want to eat. I think people could start adapting to these types of diets at the very first sign of a problem, or even just as a way to live a life to prevent these things.

We are in this battle with ever-increasing numbers of people who are struggling with mental health issues. If we could use diet as a tool, we could save a lot of people many years of misery.

Finally, I want to stress the importance of prioritizing food and health. I grew up in Nashville and love the area, but after our son was born, we chose to move away because it was too expensive. We now live in an area where we can afford to prioritize our health. We make sure that we have enough money to buy the food we need and to pay for the healthcare we need (because most of the services of naturopaths and other holistic health providers are not covered by health insurance).

We changed our whole lives to support our health.

EDITOR'S NOTES: KEY TAKEAWAYS FROM EMILY'S STORY

- Having access to the best medical care means little if that care is all conventional and focused on symptom management, rather than healing the root cause, and the ease with which the medical establishment hands out prescriptions for antidepressants and anxiolytics (including benzodiazepines) borders on malpractice.

- The impact of the Standard American Diet (ultra-processed foods high in sugars and seed oils) on childhood development can be seen in both the critical mental and physical health issues of our children, starting at a young age.

- Healthy foods and diet are a major driver for good mental health, as 95 percent of the serotonin production in the body takes place in the gut; serotonin is a critical neurotransmitter that regulates mood, reward, sleep, digestion, and other functions.

- Food is more than medicine; healthy, nutrient-dense food delivers a message to your gut microbiome and mitochondria (and the rest of your body and brain) that you value life, living, and want to live your healthiest life.

- When the foods you're eating are causing issues, you may need to experiment by process of elimination to learn which foods are best for your body, gut, and brain.

CHAPTER EIGHTEEN
Susan's Story

FROM EXHAUSTION TO VITALITY

Name: Susan Bird

How do you feel (mentally and physically) now? I feel the healthiest physically, mentally, and emotionally than at any other time in my life.

How were you (mentally and physically) before you started? Before I started this path, I was exhausted and was developing physical and mental health related issues from bad habits.

Best aspect of your plan: It doesn't feel restrictive and there are SO MANY things to eat.

Hardest part of your plan: It takes deliberate planning and preparation.

Key indicators of your health and healing: On a recent trip to see a medical provider I was told that I had the "lab results of an 18-year-old" and that the doctor wished his blood work looked like mine.

Biggest surprise of your health journey: I feel released from my negative relationship with, or attachment to, food.

I was raised on a dairy farm in rural Utah, the youngest of four. We grew and harvested 85 percent of our own food. We raised beef, pork, chicken, rabbit, corn, tomatoes, berries, beans, peas, potatoes, apples, cherries, pears, and plums. We preserved most of our own food by freezing, canning, or bottling.

My mom made amazing homemade bread every week. Ice cream and fast food were not something we had often, reserved for birthdays and holidays.

Growing up "poor," these things became an obsession to me. I distinctly remember being reprimanded for eating an entire plate of cookies at a church member's home when my mom and I were visiting. This quickly taught me that I needed to hide the foods I ate that were considered "off-limits."

This began a childhood of seeking food that I wasn't supposed to eat like Twinkies, Hostess pies, Zingers (who remembers Zingers!) and eating them to excess. As a Tomboy, I quickly gained weight.

I wouldn't have been considered obese then, but I was thicker than my siblings and any of my peers, despite constantly playing outside, riding horses, and later playing and lettering in four sports in high school.

When I was 15, my oldest sister was diagnosed with both anorexia and bulimia and was hospitalized several times. As the youngest child in a family that didn't communicate about such things, I was never informed about this period in our family history. After my sister's diagnosis, my mom took every opportunity to feed me. I was chastised for "wasting" food and was made to finish everything on my plate, even if it meant sitting at the dinner table for hours.

Thus began my tumultuous relationship with food.

Moving away from home only exacerbated the problem. I could binge eat more openly – never around my roommates, and I didn't have my mom or dad taking inventory of the fridge.

As a college athlete, I made poor nutritional decisions, and this carried over into my negative relationship with alcohol too. Looking back, I can give my younger self some grace. It was the late 1980s early 1990s and I didn't know what I know about nutrition now, even though I was a college athlete and majored in physical education!

Playing college sports heightened my problems. Being so active felt like a license to eat whatever I wanted when I wanted. Even our team meals weren't what I call nutritious by today's standards. But the theory held steady. I could eat what I wanted when I wanted for the most part, but it wasn't without constant pressure and stress from coaching staff about my weight.

I recently looked through some old photo albums and saw my driver's license from when I was 16 listed my weight as 145 lbs. Of course, we should add 5 pounds to that because I'm sure it was an under representation of what I weighed at the time.

I remember while playing volleyball at Boise State University, my coaches and trainers would reprimand me for weighing between 152-156 pounds even though

I held weight-lifting records for volleyball athletes in bench press and deadlift, had a 22-inch vertical leap, broke every single setting record that was established at the time, and was an all-conference player.

After graduation with my Bachelor of Science in Physical Education, I elected to pursue a career as a United States Marine Corps Officer. In 1995, I was selected to be one of the first women combat engineer officers. Technically this was a combat Military Occupational Specialty (MOS) at the time, so women weren't allowed in traditional combat units, or to be in combat.

Although this is the MOS I wanted, it brought the scrutiny of what seemed like the entire U.S. military. At the time, the height and weight regulations for women were incredibly difficult for a "fit" woman to meet. For my height of 5'7" I was allowed a maximum weight of 148 pounds. For the first 4 years of my career, I never fell within regulations. I received evaluations that were stellar, but always had the exception of being out of height and weight standards. Waivers at this time were few and far between and were mostly reserved for men who were 5'4", weighed 200 pounds, and were competitive body builders (as an example).

It didn't matter that I maxed (scored full points) or ran a first-class physical fitness test and could drop over half of my all-male platoon on physical training runs. The only thing that mattered was the tape and the scale. Even the measurements they used for body composition were outdated. I usually landed somewhere around 24 percent body fat, higher than the allowed 20 percent.

This scrutiny and pressure to fall within height and weight standards led to an obsession with working out; namely weight training and running. It also started an obsession with counting macro and micro calories. I spent the next 6 years of my career and life quietly being a functional anorexic. I never could get the bulimic part; I just couldn't force myself to vomit. Instead, I would spend hours in the gym.

Outside of the gym, I carried around a very large cooler that contained my food for the day. All while giving the outward appearance that I was healthy and happy.

When I deployed for two tours to Iraq in 2003 and 2004, it didn't stop me from obsessing about my fitness and my weight. It just meant that I had to manage with the food I could get, sometimes in a chow hall, sometimes sent from home.

Working out and sweating was never an issue, except for a couple of initial months in 2003 during the beginning of the Iraq War. Being on or near the front lines wasn't conducive to long runs. During my second tour, and the most stressful time of my Marine Corps career, I was simultaneously being investigated for "Don't Ask, Don't Tell" while being in the middle of a combat zone; all of my free time away from the command center was spent running or in the gym tent.

Food was merely to fuel my workouts.

I left Iraq the second time weighing 125 pounds with 7 percent body fat. Once back to the real world, the things I did while deployed to manage my stress were unsustainable. While awaiting the final outcome of my investigation, my stress response shifted back to what it was in my childhood.

I once more began to eat and drink my way through life. To cope with the stress of not knowing what would happen to the career I loved, I would stop at the liquor store and the convenience store on my way home every night and buy food and wine.

Every day I would claim I wouldn't do those things again, but I could not stop. I couldn't stop at one glass of wine, and I certainly couldn't stop at one cookie or whatever food I had decided to binge eat that day.

By the time I separated from the Marine Corps five months after returning from Iraq, I had gained nearly 60 lbs. I was the heaviest that I had ever been in my life. This was late 2005. No one talked about PTSD or trauma back then.

I continued to battle my relationship with food and alcohol, only winning occasionally. On those occasions when I thought I was winning the "weight" war, other parts of my life suffered; relationships, family, work.

Whenever I felt like I was winning the weight war, it was usually due to some type of extreme measure. I've done a raw diet, I've ran ultra-marathons, and have gone to unsustainable lengths to incorporate fitness routines into my day, solely to stay ahead of the weight gain.

Some of those unsustainable lengths included food prep that takes an entire day and waking up at 4 a.m. to work out before my workday starts at 7 a.m. It wasn't until 2015, ten years after leaving the military, that I decided to seek the mental health care that I didn't know I needed.

My drinking and lifestyle were taking its toll on my mind and body. I quit drinking alcohol (which saved my life), I met my current partner who has supported me unconditionally throughout my journey, and I began researching alternative therapeutic modalities such as psychedelic plant medicines to face, address, and process trauma.

In 2023, a friend recommended that I investigate a veteran organization that focuses on helping disabled veterans heal through plant medicine therapies. After being accepted to one of their medicinal retreats, part of the program included adhering to a strict diet protocol. This would ensure participants could get the maximum benefits from the plant medicine, ayahuasca.

I began cutting out some foods before the specified timeline, including fast foods, processed foods, and red meat. I immediately lost 10 pounds and noticed that the menopause symptoms that I had been having were less severe.

Once I was in the diet restriction timeline and was adhering to it, I lost another 10 pounds. Prior to departing for the retreat, I noticed that all my menopause symptoms were gone. These included migraines (1-2 per week), hot flashes, mood swings, sleeplessness, indigestion, and body aches.

I felt more in tune to my body than I had felt in years. My flexibility improved. My ability to focus improved. My relationship improved.

After going through an incredibly healing yet difficult journey on the retreat, I found that food didn't consume my thoughts. I wasn't obsessing over my weight and instead I was listening to my body.

In the past, I have had conversations with therapists and counselors about how some people find it possible to listen to what their body needs. I didn't buy into it. I thought it was impossible for me.

Since my return from the retreat, I haven't strayed far from the prescribed diet. I'm still listening to my body. But, aside from all the amazing benefits that I have experienced, the most amazing part for me is that I no longer have the desire to overeat or binge on food.

Since transitioning from my old diet and eating habits, I have effectively eliminated red meats, dairy, and most processed foods. I have yet to re-introduce caffeine; I went from two cups of coffee per day to two cups of tea, and then completely eliminated caffeine earlier this year.

I also eliminated my Adderall prescription at the same time and I don't feel like I am less productive without it.

My food choices mainly consist of fresh fruits, vegetables, and fish or poultry. I have found some amazing recipes for almond flour bread and almond flour muffins, which are delicious, and contain 6 grams of protein per slice.

I use honey or monk fruit sweetener, if I use any sweetener at all.

As someone who grew up on a dairy farm drinking unpasteurized milk, I find that almond or oat milk tastes much better and doesn't leave me feeling congested or too full. I have enjoyed making my own salad dressing, finding a recipe that I like, and tweaking it to my tastes. My current favorites are cilantro lime dressing or lemon vinaigrette.

I have also enjoyed using mushrooms as a source of protein, and love to season and sauté shitakes or portobellos. Grilled lion's mane is also delicious, but slightly more difficult to find without hitting up a farmers market.

I can be a creature of habit and eat the same foods for several days, but I have been able to rotate through a few favorites over the course of a week to keep things interesting, rotating through salmon, chicken, or a plant-based protein.

For sweets or snacks, I have turned to some Trader Joe's staples, such as plantain chips, chocolate covered pistachios, dried mango mini rice cakes, dried fruit, nuts, and an oat-milk-based ice cream.

My partner is ecstatic that we actually have snacks in the house. Before this health journey, I would have eaten all of what we had in one sitting. Now I don't feel the need to do that, which feels incredible.

I'm able to eat what my body needs and then stop. I can have just one cookie or snack. I enjoy cooking again, and exploring a whole new world of foods and recipes that I wouldn't have otherwise.

I can focus on me and my healing without letting food or the way I feel about my weight get in the way of that healing, and for that I am grateful.

EDITOR'S NOTES: KEY TAKEAWAYS FROM SUSAN'S STORY

- As parents, it is so important to carefully explain food guidelines and health with children so that they don't learn to hide food or to consider some foods as "off limits."
- Family upbringing can have such a lasting, lifelong effect on adult behaviors and relationships with food.
- Some institutions place too much emphasis on health and weight requirements, which only puts more pressure on people and can lead to an obsession with controlling weight. The key should always be a focus on health and nutrition, not weight or body mass index (BMI).
- Often trauma fuels our bad relationships with food (and other substances), which is why it is so important to heal old trauma wounds, to do both a health and healing journey.

CHAPTER NINETEEN
Shilpa's Story

FARASHA

Name: Shilpa Kudekar

How do you feel (mentally and physically) now? Serene and strong.

How were you (mentally and physically) before you started? Miserable and weak.

Best aspect of your plan: Cultivating a healthy mindset.

Hardest part of your plan: Sticking to a healthy mindset.

Key indicators of your health and healing: Measurement (Inches), biomarkers, mental/emotional health, and fitness level (strength and endurance).

Biggest surprise of your health journey: Discovering my "Ikigai," my purpose, my passion: Reiki.

(*Farasha* means butterfly in Arabic language; it's a metaphor for transformation.)

I have always had a sweet tooth as far as I can remember.

Growing up in India, food was life, especially the delicious melt-in-your-mouth traditional sweets. Being young, I thought I could overcome anything, but what I didn't realize is that life happens.

At the age of 18, I left home to go to Australia. I had found my sense of freedom.

The first thing I did was eat a hamburger and drink a milkshake.

You see, back in India, Mum made everything at home – including street food. All of it was healthy and tasty! She made her own butter, ghee, curd, masalas, pickles, chutneys, dressings, sauces, savory and sweet treats…everything from scratch.

We never ate junk.

I was utterly fascinated by the commercials on TV showing all the yummy foods but never got a chance to eat them. Both my parents were into a holistic lifestyle. Wellness was akin to a mantra for those two. They lived and breathed it; day in and day out. Mum and Dad instilled the same values in my brother and me.

Yet when I was in Australia, I gave in to temptation! I started eating junk food and drinking alcohol. Idleness set in and comfort food just got too comfortable to the point that I started changing, not just physically, but mentally and emotionally too.

I was still salvageable at university, as walking and dancing kept me active and somewhat fit. But, when I joined the workforce, all bets were off!

As a medical scientist in a rural lab, I was doing a lot of on-call work, which resulted in many broken sleeps and the worst eating patterns (that turned into habits!!).

I ate whatever I could lay my hands on. Sugars and carbs were my best friends. From sweetened cereals, pasta, pizza, chips and gravy, fairy bread, cookies, blocks of chocolates with big bowls of ice cream, I devoured them all!!

By the time I realized it, I had put on a lot of weight. I was stiff and lethargic. My body was sore, my mind was hazy and foggy, and my emotions were on a rollercoaster ride.

My health had slowly started to deteriorate. I was getting a lot of heartburn, acidity, reflux, muscle aches and cramps, lower back pain and cold. I got bloodwork done that did not look promising especially for my liver, kidneys, and pancreas, as their functions were impaired, while my hormones were all over the place.

I also got an imaging test done that showed I had a hiatal hernia (later on I found out that my lower esophageal sphincter was weak and would not close completely). This meant I could no longer have big portions nor eat spicy and fried meals. I was mad. I did not like myself one bit; actually, I did not like what I had become... angry, impatient, lazy, unhappy, volatile.

I had reached a point where I thought everything was too hard and I simply wanted to give up. This saddened my family. How did I get to this point in my life? I was very healthy and fit as a child and as a teenager. Where did I go wrong? Why did I let myself go?

I wanted to leave and start somewhere fresh, not realizing that change starts from within – until it was a bit too late. But more on that a little later!

To fulfill that need, I applied for work all over the globe, until one day I received an offer from a world-class healthcare facility in the UAE.

Before making my way to Abu Dhabi, I had a one-month stopover in India to see my family. My Mum took one look at me and decided to take charge. She made me eat only healthy homemade meals. I wasn't allowed to look at any other food or even think about it...

I stopped eating fried foods and refined carbs, so no rice, bread, pasta, chips, – basically anything white. I went for walks with my Dad, who encouraged me to get back into exercising, starting with active recovery.

My parents were my pillars of strength and hope. They supported me through all my ordeals. Mum and Dad kept saying to me "*Mind over matter my darling, take baby steps but keep going forward and never give up. You can do this.*"

After saying our goodbyes, we flew to our new home in the beautiful sandy oasis. Throughout the travel, I kept reminiscing about my past, debating my old eating ways in Australia. I knew no good was going to come out of that and I had to let go so I could move on, but definitely learn from those experiences.

Guess what? Life happened and I was tasked with setting up a new laboratory, which was challenging, yet also a lot of fun. The honeymoon period was over when the hospital opened up and was fully operational.

Doing shift work played havoc on my mental and physical well-being. I kept going by eating small healthy meals. However, I was also gulping down cheesecakes, and here I thought I was doing well with my food but I could not understand why I didn't feel better?! (I didn't make the connection that sugars equal carbs until late in the game.)

When my Dad passed away unexpectedly in 2017, that trauma took me back to square one with my eating habits. I literally ate my feelings by downing entire packets of biscuits, chocolates, and tubs of ice cream.

That continued until one day my Mum looked at me point blank and said "*If you don't stop now and take charge of your life, you are going to be lying six feet under pretty soon.*"

Her statement shocked me, but I wasn't surprised, as Mum was always brutally honest!

The consequence of my actions screwed my body immensely. I was very sick and my biomarkers were abnormal – we are talking about high levels of HbA1C, triglycerides, liver enzymes, creatinine. I ended up having fatty liver, diminished kidney function, reduced insulin sensitivity, and a banged up hormonal profile.

All in all, I was heading toward metabolic syndrome.

I remember my doctor telling me, *"I am not going to give you any meds, so change your lifestyle through holistic interventions. Come and see me in four months."*

That day, as I walked out of her office, I decided that enough was enough, and that I was going to change and take charge of my life.

It was like ripping a band-aid off.

The first thing I did was study articles on the ketogenic diet. The question was, how do I apply this knowledge? Where do I start? The only way I could think of was 'Self-Experimentation'! I kicked things off by measuring myself, another factor to add to my baseline, besides my horrifying biomarkers. I looked up recipes and started cooking with my husband, which I quite enjoyed!

It was through the process of elimination, trial and error, that I figured out what worked for me. For example; I realized that consuming dairy, legumes, and whole grains made me gassy! I was constantly bloated and my gut wasn't happy Whereas, eating grass-fed beef and whole eggs made my skin soft and supple, I also felt stronger. Also, munching on an array of colorful vegetables and fruits enhanced my immune system, and I did not get colds too often!

This was utterly fascinating to me!!

I was becoming more and more aware of ingredients. Physically, I felt great; mentally, very clear; and emotionally, well balanced. I lost 25kgs and quite a lot of inches, especially from my waistline! Oh, it was so good to see all that weight melt off and those love handles disappear!! But, in the midst of this, I also lost a lot of muscle mass, and that made me look gaunt. So, I started doing Yoga and Pilates. I believe these exercises centered me, brought me stability and built my strength. At this point in my life, I got back into practicing Reiki for self-care. (I wanted to be at peace…the one thing I truly desired.)

After four months, I went back to my GP and got my labs done. We tested the same biomarkers again. The results were incredible. My comprehensive metabolic panel was normal! I was very happy that I could get to this moment in my life.

I told Mum about my achievement. She was over the moon with pride and joy. Now the challenging part was sustaining this newfound way of life. It wasn't impossible, but was it difficult…hell yes! I pushed past the temptations by being disciplined and consistent.

Unfortunately, this happy journey came to a sudden halt when my Mum tragically passed away in 2019. It felt like my whole world had suddenly ended…I couldn't breathe, sleep, think... I was stuck in a nightmarish loop of constant fear and panic, with no closure nor any relief in sight.

I was at the lowest point in my life where I was ready to throw all the hard work down the drain and drown my sorrows in the sugary sweets and carb-loaded foods that looked so very delicious. I was coveting them...especially alcohol.

My brother and my husband saw the desperation on my face. I vaguely remember both of them saying *"Please don't go back; mum was so proud of you."* I could see the plea in my brother's eyes. I realized then that I needed to be strong for us, that I wouldn't give up nor give in.

What gave me solace was my discipline and consistency with food.

I delved into nutrient-dense, polyphenol-rich vegetables and fruits ('Eat the Rainbow' – I understood this term a little later in my exploration), grass-fed or pasture-raised meat and poultry, nuts and seeds, lard, cold pressed extra virgin olive oil, organic raw extra virgin coconut oil, dark chocolate, spices, herbs, and fermented foods.

I believe I had only scratched the surface...there was so much more to unearth!

So, I kept on searching until I stumbled upon an amazing TEDx talk by Dr. Terry Wahls. This incredible soul had reversed her symptoms of MS solely through lifestyle interventions! She was my "Wonder Woman" and still is to this day. Dr. Wahls made me realize that "Food is information, Food is medicine."

This was a game-changer for me. It gave me hope!

Then, the pandemic hit!! Throughout this period, I kept going strong with my commitment to nutrition. This increased my thirst for knowledge, so I kept digging for more information and came across 'Keto-biotic diet, Evolutionary food, Gut microbiome, Prebiotics, Probiotics, Nutrient Bioavailability, Intermittent fasting, Mitochondrial health, Supplements, Blue zones'...and a whole lot more!!

Now this blew my mind.

I learned that nutrition wasn't simply about eating healthy; it was also about: How you prepare the food? What time you eat the food? What order you eat the food in? What region do the ingredients come from? What kind of farming style/practice is used to cultivate the crops? What kind of soil the crops are grown in? Is the soil clean or contaminated? Did the grazers turn the topsoil over?... The list goes on and on!

Furthermore, my discoveries led me to Dr. Mark Hyman, Dr. William Li, Dr. Rhonda Patrick, Dr. Sara Gottfried, Dr. Andrew Huberman, Dr. Peter Attia, and Dr. Mindy Pelz. Reading their books and articles as well as listening to their podcasts gave me an insight into the world of Functional Medicine. This new understanding upped the ante and changed the dynamics of the game completely. I knew I had a lot of work ahead of me.

I wanted to grow and evolve. My curiosity led me to 'Institute for Functional Medicine – Functional Medicine Coaching Academy' where I completed the one-year health coaching program.

Last February I graduated and became a Functional Medicine Certified Health Coach.

It was then that I realized that even though I had maintained my discipline with food, I still had a long way to go in terms of achieving and enhancing my overall well-being.

To reach my goal, I knew I had to look into exercising and mindfulness. Besides walking and doing Yoga and Pilates, I also started attending HIIT, dance fitness, strength and conditioning, and kickboxing classes at my hospital gym. I gained a lot of muscle mass and as a consequence, lost quite a bit of body fat. I got toned, I got fit!

This process made me realize that it's all about *mindset, what your mind believes your body achieves.* To etch this thinking, I kept on practicing and sharing Reiki, my "Ikigai," my purpose for being. It made me feel tranquil. What aligned my physical, emotional, and mental wellness was Reiki.

To date, discipline, commitment, and mindset have helped me maintain my overall well-being. I only eat fresh, organic, polyphenol-rich, grass-fed, and nutrient-dense foods. I do intermittent fasting and my workouts include a mixture of endurance and resistance training.

I have started chanting, meditating, and doing breathwork, along with heat shock therapy (steam sauna). I am going to jump into an ice bath soon for some cold shock treatment and then, perhaps move on to cryotherapy. I am really excited and happy!! For once, I am looking forward to a bright future.

What keeps me thriving is my gratitude for life and its teachings, my passion for Reiki, and my love for my gorgeous patients, their families, and my awesome caregivers. This journey truly has been humbling, gratifying, and transformational.

Shilpa is a clinical instructor for Point of Care Testing (POCT) and has been with Cleveland Clinic Abu Dhabi (CCAD) for 10 years. Her passion for wellness led Shilpa to study and graduate from Functional Medicine Coaching Academy; Institute for Functional Medicine (FMCA; IFM) in 2023 and is now a Functional Medicine Certified Health Coach. She recently completed her Advanced Sound Alchemy train-

ing and is now a Sound Healing Practitioner. Shilpa has been on a lifelong journey with Reiki and as an intuitive Reiki Master Practitioner of 25 years. You can connect with her on LinkedIn: linkedin.com/in/shilpa-kudekar-mcneilly-a92ab939

EDITOR'S NOTES: KEY TAKEAWAYS FROM SHILPA'S STORY

- Even with an upbringing that focused on healthy and homemade foods, the lure from food marketer's commercials is too strong, encouraging people to eat their ultra-processed, imposter foods.

- Working long hours, perhaps with a bit of workaholism, can lead to eating only convenience foods – and especially foods that offer "comfort" in the form of sugar and carbohydrates.

- Unhealthy diets can have both mental and physical health consequences. Physically, gaining weight, bloating, brain fog. Mentally, depression, anxiety, anger, impatience, volatile behaviors.

- It's never too late to start a health journey – or to restart one. The key to finding health is experimenting with all the real, nutrient-dense foods available to you to discover that unique blend of foods that are *best for you* – that make you feel good/healthy mentally and physically.

PART FOUR: HEALING REVOLUTION RESOURCES

 INSPIRING QUOTE

"If I could give one tip for people – it's not an exercise or nutrition regimen. It's to walk your talk and believe in yourself, because at the end of the day, the dumbbell and diet don't get you in shape. It's your accountability to your word." — Brett Hoebel

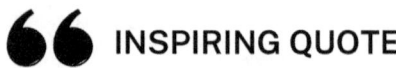 **INSPIRING QUOTE**

"The lack of access to proper nutrition is not only fueling obesity, it is leading to food insecurity and hunger among our children." — Tom Vilsack

Healing Revolution Diet: Health, Nutrition, and Diet Resources

HEALTH, NUTRITION, AND DIET DOCUMENTARIES

A Place at the Table (2012): Investigates incidents of hunger and food insecurity experienced by millions of Americans, and proposed solutions to the problem.

Beyond Food (2017): explores the ways a group of extraordinary people live amazing lives, eat delicious food while extracting more energy and mental focus from their daily rituals.

Bite Size (2014): Tells the stories of 4 kids around the country as they embark on a journey to become healthier and lose weight.

Deadly Obesity Epidemic (2019): Delves deep into the growing health crisis of obesity. It examines the causes, consequences, and potential solutions related to this chronic disease.

Diet Fiction (2019): Exposes the most popular diets on the planet as well as several misconceptions about weight loss and nutrition, and includes filmmaker Michal Siewierski's dieting journey.

Fat Fiction (2020): Leading health experts examine the history of the U.S. Dietary Guidelines and question decades of dietary advice insisting that saturated fats are bad for our health.

FAT: A Documentary (2019): Health expert Vinnie Tortorich exposes the history behind widespread myths and lies regarding healthy eating, fat, and weight loss.

Fed Up (2014): Examines America's obesity epidemic and the food industry's role in aggravating it, including that far more people get sick from what they eat than previously realized.

Food Fight (2008): Discusses how American agricultural policy and food culture developed in the 20th century, and how the California food movement rebelled against big agribusiness to launch the local organic food movement.

Food, Inc. (2008): Provides an unflattering look inside America's corporate greed-controlled food industry, demonstrating that it is unhealthy, unethical, and environmentally harmful. Game-changer.

Hungry for Change (2012): Exposes shocking secrets the diet, weight loss and food industries don't want you to know about deceptive strategies designed to keep you coming back for more.

Killer at Large (2008): Delves into the politics, social effects, and problems associated with the rising epidemic of American obesity.

King Corn (2007): Follows two college friends investigating the role of government subsidies in encouraging the huge amount of corn grown, while showing how most foods contain corn in some form.

Kiss the Ground (2020): Explores regenerative agriculture as a solution to the climate crisis. By regenerating the world's soils, we can stabilize Earth's climate, restore ecosystems, and create abundant food supplies.

The Magic Pill (2017): Follows doctors, patients, scientists, chefs, farmers, and journalists from around the globe – showing how people are combating illness by embracing fat as the main fuel.

Rotten (2018-19): A compelling docuseries that dives deeply into the food production underworld to expose the corruption, waste, and real dangers behind every day eating habits.

Sacred Cow (2021): Well-managed cows raised on regenerative farms is the focus examining the fundamental moral, environmental, and nutritional quandaries faced in raising and eating animals.

Sugar Coated (2015): Explores the impact on human health of the heavy use of sugar and how the food industry sugar-coated science, sweetened the food supply, and seduced a planet, one spoonful at a time.

Super Size Me (2004): While examining the influence of the fast food industry, filmmaker Morgan Spurlock explores the consequences on his health of a diet of solely McDonald's food for one month.

Symphony of the Soil (2013): An artistic exploration of the miraculous substance called soil and the elaborate relationships and mutuality between soil, water, the atmosphere, plants, and animals.

That Sugar Film (2014): Showcases an experiment on the effects of a high sugar diet on a healthy body, from foods commonly perceived as healthy, and explores where sugar lurks on supermarket shelves.

What The Health (2017): Uncovers possibly the largest health secret of our time and the collusion among industry, government, pharmaceutical, and health organizations in keeping this information from us.

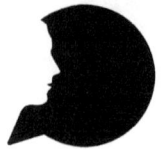

AUTHOR INSIGHT

Nutritionists have long classified the key macronutrients in food as proteins, fats, and carbohydrates. But because fiber plays such an important role with the gut microbiome and overall health, I consider it a fourth macronutrient that should be included in our daily diet.

HEALTH, NUTRITION, AND DIET BOOKS

Animal, Vegetable, Miracle: Our Year of Seasonal Eating, by Barbara Kingsolver, with Steven L. Hopp and Camile Kingsolver. (2008) Inspired by the flavors and culinary arts of a local food culture, they explore many a farmers market and diversified organic farms, showing us how to put food back at the center of the political and family agenda. ISBN: 0571233570

The Ancestral Diet Revolution: How Vegetable Oils and Processed Foods Destroy Our Health - and How to Recover! by Chris A Knobbe, MD, and Suzanne J Alexander, M.Ed. (2023) Makes the point that the single most important component of an ancestral diet is the elimination of vegetable oils, which are highly pro-oxidative, pro-inflammatory, toxic, and nutrient deficient. ISBN: 1734071761

Brain Maker: The Power of Gut Microbes to Heal and Protect Your Brain - for Life, by Dr. David Perlmutter with Kristin Loberg. Explains the interplay between intestinal microbes and the brain, describing how the microbiome develops from birth and evolves based on the environment, and how nurturing gut health through a few easy strategies can alter your brain s destiny for the better. ISBN: 1473619351

Can It & Ferment It: More Than 75 Satisfying Small-Batch Canning and Fermentation Recipes for the Whole Year, by Stephanie Thurow. (2017) Explains the differences between the canning and fermentation processes, emphasizes the importance of using local and organic produce, describes canning and fermenting terminology. ISBN: 1510717420

Change Your Diet, Change Your Mind: A Powerful Plan to Improve Mood, Overcome Anxiety, and Protect Memory for a Lifetime of Optimal Mental Health, by Georgia Ede, MD. (2024) Combines the surprising truth about brain food with the cutting-edge science of brain metabolism to achieve extraordinary improvements to your emotional, cognitive, and physical health. ISBN: 1538739070

Cultured Food for Health: A Guide to Healing Yourself with Probiotic Foods Kefir, Kombucha, Cultured Vegetables, by Donna Schwenk. (2015) Focusing on the notion that all disease begins in the gut – a claim made by Hippocrates, the father of medicine – the author brings together cutting-edge research to highlight the links between an imbalanced microbiome and a host of ailments. ISBN: 1401947832

Cu-RE Your Fatigue: The Root Cause and How To Fix It On Your Own, by Morley Robbins. (2021) Designed for those seeking the truth in human metabolism and Metabolic Syndrome, and those wanting to take back control of their health. It is one part textbook and one part user's guide based on a decade of research and client experience. ISBN: 1662910282

Dark Calories: How Vegetable Oils Destroy Our Health and How We Can Get It Back, by Catherine Shanahan, MD. (2024) Explains how eight common seed oils cause the cellular damage that underlies virtually all chronic disease, exposes the corruption that deceives doctors and consumers alike, and gives readers a clear roadmap to recovery and rejuvenation. ISBN: 0306832399

Dirty Genes: A Breakthrough Program to Treat the Root Cause of Illness and Optimize Your Health, by Dr. Ben Lynch. (2020) Genes can be "born dirty" or merely "act dirty" in response to environment, diet, or lifestyle – causing lifelong, life-threatening, and chronic health problems – showing how dirty genes can be cleaned up with targeted and personalized plans. ISBN: 006269815X

Eat Dirt: Why Leaky Gut May Be the Root Cause of Your Health Problems and 5 Surprising Steps to Cure It, by Dr. Josh Axe. (2017) Starved of actual nutrition and overtaxed by chemicals, stress, and excessive antimicrobial use, we are developing microscopic tears in our intestinal walls, which can lead to a condition known as "leaky gut syndrome." ISBN: 0062433679

Eat to Beat Disease: The New Science of How Your Body Can Heal Itself, by William W. Li, MD. (2019) Learn how to identify the strategies and dosages for using food to transform your resilience and health, showcasing 200+ health-boosting foods that can starve cancer, reduce the risk of dementia, and beat dozens of avoidable diseases. ISBN: 1538714620

8 Weeks to Optimum Health: A Proven Program for Taking Full Advantage of Your Body's Natural Healing Power, by Andrew Weil, MD. (2008). A classic from one of the most respected doctors, and that covers diet, exercise, lifestyle, stress, and environment issues, all aspects of daily living that affect health and well-being, with a focus on prevention. ISBN: 034549802X

Fiber Fueled: The Plant-Based Gut Health Program for Losing Weight, Restoring Your Health, and Optimizing Your Microbiome, by Will Bulsiewicz, MD. (2020) Gut health is the key to boosting metabolism, balancing hormones, and taming the inflammation that causes a host of diseases. Discusses best ways to fuel our guts is with dietary fiber. ISBN: 059308456X

Food Fix: How to Save Our Health, Our Economy, Our Communities, and Our Planet - One Bite at a Time, by Mark Hyman, MD. (2021) Explains how our food and agriculture policies are corrupted by money and lobbies that drive our biggest global crises: the spread of obesity and food-related chronic disease, climate change, poverty, violence, educational achievement gaps, and more. ISBN: 0316453145

Forever Strong: A New, Science-Based Strategy for Aging Well, by Dr. Gabrielle Lyon. (2023) Learn how to reboot your metabolism, build strength, and extend your life with this new guidebook that demonstrates the importance of muscle for health and longevity. The book offers an easy-to-follow food, fitness, and self-care program ISBN: 1668007878

Good Energy: The Surprising Connection Between Metabolism and Limitless Health, by Casey Means, MD, with Calley Means. (2004) Nearly every health problem we face can be explained by how well the cells in our body create and use energy. Discover why we need our cells to be optimally powered so that they can create "good energy." ISBN: 0593712641

Gut Check: Unleash the Power of Your Microbiome to Reverse Disease and Transform Your Mental, Physical, and Emotional Health, by Steven R Gundry, MD. (2004) Reveals the emerging science proving that Hippocrates was right that all disease begins in the gut. When our microbiomes are out of balance, it affects our many aspects of our physical and mental health. ISBN: 0062911775

Healthy Gut, Healthy You: The Personalized Plan to Transform Your Health from the Inside Out, by Dr. Michael Ruscio. (2018) This book shows how modern lifestyle changes and the widespread use of antibiotics have made our guts more vulnerable than ever before. The good news is that almost any ailment can be healed, but only by treating the root cause; the gut. ISBN: 0999766805

The Holistic Guide to Gut Health: Discover the Truth About Leaky Gut, Balancing Your Microbiome, and Restoring Whole-Body Health, by Dr. Mark Stengler. (2024) A comprehensive yet accessible approach to healing leaky gut and the many uncomfortable symptoms it causes. Whole-body health can be restored with this integrative program, which includes prebiotic and probiotic recipes. ISBN: 1401975100

The Holistic Guide to Wellness : Herbal Protocols for Common Ailments, by Nicole Apelian, Ph.D. (2023) Includes healing protocols for chronic pain, GERD and acid reflux, Parkinson's disease, type-2 diabetes, leaky gut, lupus, Lyme disease, multiple sclerosis, parasites, candida, bacterial infections, psoriasis and eczema, tinnitus, osteoporosis, thyroid, and many more. ISBN: 1735481580

Holistic Homesteading: A Guide to a Sustainable and Regenerative Lifestyle, by Roxanne Ahern. (2022) Provides the tools for living slowly, intentionally, and better through permaculture, edible gardening, and organic farming – for both new and seasoned homesteaders, including advice for retrofitting urban and suburban lifestyles and landscapes to shift toward sustainability. ISBN: 1642509957

How Not to Die: Discover the Foods Scientifically Proven to Prevent and Reverse Disease, by Michael Greger, MD, FACLM, with Gene Stone. (2015) The founder of NutritionFacts.org examines the fifteen top causes of premature death in America and explains how nutritional and lifestyle interventions can be better than prescription pills and other medical procedures. ISBN: 1250066115

Intermittent Fasting for Everyone: Unlock the Power of Time-Restricted Eating, by Murad Murad. (2024) Are you ready to transform your health, boost your energy, and achieve your wellness goals? Dive into the definitive guide on intermittent fasting and discover the secrets of this revolutionary eating pattern that has taken the health and fitness world by storm. ISBN: 979-8328992435

Just One Heart: A Cardiologist's Guide to Healing, Health, and Happiness, by Jonathan Fisher M.D. (2024) Empowers readers with simple tools and daily practices to manage stress, cultivate lasting joy, and connect with what truly matters. The book is filled with lessons learned from the author's own struggles through anxiety and burnout, inspiring patient stories, and more. ISBN: 1636760007

Keto Metabolic Breakthrough: A Radical Approach to Reversing Metabolic Dysfunction, Optimizing Nutrient Timing, and Balancing Hormones for Success on a Low-Carb Diet, by David Jockers, DNM, DC. (2021) Using the principles of the low-carb, high-fat ketogenic diet, the author shows how to remedy metabolic dysfunction by changing one's metabolic state. ISBN: 1628603674

Make Food Simple: Take the Stress and Confusion Out of Nutrition And Make Quick, Healthy Meals For the Entire Family, by Dr. Blake Livingood with Jessica Livingood. (2019) Did you know that 90 percent of disease is driven by our lifestyle choices, especially what we put on our dinner plate? Find nutrient-dense, quick, and healthy recipes for meals for the entire family. ISBN: 057851091X

Metabolical: The Lure and the Lies of Processed Food, Nutrition and Modern Medicine: Unpacking the Science Behind Food and Health, Robert H Lustig, MD, MSL. (2021) Makes the case that food is the only lever we have to effect biochemical change to improve our health, stating all eating should be based on two novel criteria: protect the liver and feed the gut. ISBN: 0063027712

The Nourished Kitchen: Farm-to-Table Recipes for the Traditional Foods Lifestyle Featuring Bone Broths, Fermented Vegetables, Grass-Fed Meats, Wholesome Fats, Raw Dairy, and Kombuchas, by Jennifer McGruther. (2014) An approach to cooking, fermenting, and eating that emphasizes nutrient-dense, real food over the convenience of processed, additive-laden food products. ISBN: 1607744686

Outlive: The Science and Art of Longevity, by Peter Attia, MD, with Bill Gifford. (2023) In this operating manual for longevity, Dr. Peter Attia draws on the latest science to deliver innovative nutritional interventions, techniques for optimizing exercise and sleep, and tools for addressing emotional and mental health. ISBN: 0593236599

The Probiotic Diet: Improve Digestion, Boost Your Brain Health, and Supercharge Your Immune System, by Dr. Jordan Rubin with Dr. Josh Axe and Joseph Brasco, MD. (2023) Learn how to prepare easy, delicious "gut friendly" probiotic meals, reduce common digestive symptoms such as gas, bloating, indigestion, heartburn, constipation, and diarrhea. ISBN: 0768472229

The Science-Backed Anti-Inflammatory Diet for Beginners: A Hassle-Free Guide and Simple Meal Plan To Enhance Immunity, Optimize Gut Health, and Reduce Chronic Pain at Any Age, by Yasmine Elamir, MD, and William Grist, MD. (2023) The first thirty pages discusses inflammatory foods and the rest of the book includes healthy, anti-inflammatory recipes and a three-week meal plan. Includes recipes for smoothies, meals, and more. ISBN: 979-8867732806

Smarter Not Harder: The Biohacker's Guide to Getting the Body and Mind You Want, by Dave Asprey. (2023) The master of biohacking exposes the surprising secrets of your body's operating system that is naturally designed to be lazy, which is why sweaty exercise routines and rigid diets produce such limited effects. Asprey shows readers how to conquer their operating system. ISBN: 006320472X.

Super Gut: A Four Week Plan to Reprogram Your Microbiome, Restore Health, and Lose Weight, by William Davis, MD. (2022) The ancient bacteria that keep our digestion moving have been dying, replaced by harmful microbes that don't keep us physically and mentally fit. Learn how to eliminate bad bacteria and bring back the "good" bacteria. ISBN: 0306846969

Why We Get Sick: The Hidden Epidemic at the Root of Most Chronic Disease–and How to Fight It, by Benjamin Bikman, PhD. (2021) Reveals the groundbreaking evidence linking many major diseases, including cancer, diabetes, and Alzheimer's disease, to a common root cause – insulin resistance – and shares an easy, effective plan to reverse and prevent it. ISBN: 1953295770

Young Forever: The Secrets to Living Your Longest, Healthiest Life, by Mark Hyman, MD. (2023) The author challenges us to reimagine our biology, health, and the process of aging. The book explores the biological hallmarks of aging, their causes, and their consequences – then shows how to overcome them with simple dietary, lifestyle, and emerging longevity strategies. ISBN: 0316453188

HEALTH, NUTRITION, AND FOOD EXPERTS TO FOLLOW ON SOCIAL MEDIA

(You may find them on LinkedIn, Facebook, Instagram, or X)

- Dr. Robert Lustig
- Jack Wolfson, DO
- Kristie Leong MD
- Chris Palmer, MD
- Dr. Daryl Gioffre
- Frank Lipman MD
- Bret Scher, MD
- Beth Frates MD
- Casey Means, MD
- Cate Shanahan, MD
- Paul Saladino, MD
- Lori Shemek, PhD
- Frank Lipman, MD
- Dr. Eric Berg
- Georgia Ede, MD
- Sara Gottfried, MD

- Mary Claire Haver, MD
- Jonathan Fisher, MD, FACC
- Andrew Weil, MD
- Nina Teicholz, PhD
- Dr. James DiNicolantonio
- Dr. Ben Lynch

HEALTH, NUTRITION, FOOD, AND DIET WEBSITES

- **American Community Gardening Association:** its mission is to build community by increasing and enhancing community gardening and greening across the United States and Canada. URL: https://www.communitygarden.org/
- **American Grassfed Association:** communicates the value of grassfed products to consumers, chefs, and the media and serves as a resource for information. We also advocate and work to make positive change in policies for pasture-based producers. URL: https://www.americangrassfed.org/
- **Big Green:** helping people grow their own food — with garden-based education, scalable, modular garden products and systems, and a community of support and collaboration. URL: https://biggreen.org/
- **Center for Food as Medicine:** aims to bridge the gap between traditional medicine and the use of food as medicine in the prevention, treatment, and management of disease while also increasing access to these treatments, thereby creating a more equitable food system. URL: https://foodmedcenter.org/
- **Green America:** its mission is to harness economic power – the strength of consumers, investors, businesses, and the marketplace – to create a socially just and environmentally sustainable society, including regenerative agriculture. URL: https://www.greenamerica.org/
- **Kiss the Ground:** its mission is to awaken people to the possibilities of regeneration, promoting regeneration and healthy soil as a viable solution for our wellness, water, and climate crisis. URL: https://kisstheground.com/
- **The Organic Center:** a trusted resource for scientific reporting on agriculture and food, serving up unbiased scientific findings in distilled bites so visitors can make more informed decisions, and protect wild places and biodiversity through environmentally friendly farming. URL: https://www.organic-center.org/

- **Organic Facts:** a source for unbiased and reliable information on organic and healthy food, making it easy for people to find information on all aspects of wellness and clean living. URL: https://www.organicfacts.net/
- **Organic Voices:** devoted to telling the story of organic agriculture and food production with the hope of instilling the peace of mind that going organic gives, cultivating a better understanding of what being organic really means and the environmental and health benefits choosing organic provides. URL: https://www.organicvoices.org/
- **Regeneration International:** Promoting, facilitating, and accelerating the global transition to regenerative food, farming and land management for the purpose of restoring climate stability, ending world hunger and rebuilding deteriorated social, ecological and economic systems. URL: https://regenerationinternational.org/
- **Regenerative Organic Alliance:** is a revolutionary new certification for food, textiles, and personal care ingredients. Regenerative Organic Certified farms and products meet the highest standards in the world for soil health, animal welfare, and farmworker fairness. URL: https://regenorganic.org/
- **Rodale Institute:** Conducts independent research to uncover and share regenerative organic farming practices that restore soil health, fight climate change, and fix the food system. URL: https://rodaleinstitute.org/
- **Healthline:** covers all facets of physical and mental health openly and objectively because the site is designed for the whole person – for your whole life – cutting through the confusion with straightforward, expert-reviewed, person-first experiences. URL: https://www.healthline.com/
- **America's Healthy Food Financing Initiative:** provides grants, loans, and technical assistance to improve access to healthy food in underserved areas, create and preserve quality jobs, and revitalize low-income communities. URL: https://www.investinginfood.com/
- **Action for Healthy Kids:** helps create healthier schools by bringing all the members of a school community together and equipping them with the tools and resources they need to make change happen. URL: https://www.actionforhealthykids.org/
- **Big Green:** helps people grow their own food with school and home-based programs, improving nutrition security, helping with mental health, and reconnecting people to nature. URL: https://biggreen.org/

- **Chef Ann Foundation:** helps schools serve fresh, healthy, scratch-cooked food because all children need access to fresh, healthy, delicious food. URL: https://www.chefannfoundation.org/
- **Eat Real:** nourishes the future of American kids by putting real food on the table at school, at home, and in local and national policy. Supervises a K-12 certification program designed to make eating at school not just nutritious, but delicious. URL: https://eatreal.org/
- **Farms for Life:** a Seattle-area nonprofit working to support local farmers, reduce on-farm waste, and increase access to healthy produce for underserved communities. URL: https://www.farmsforlife.org/
- **Feeding America:** ending hunger by partnering with food banks, food pantries, and local food programs to bring food to people facing hunger. We advocate for policies that create long-term solutions to hunger. URL: https://www.feedingamerica.org/
- **The Food Dignity Movement:** fights to shine a light on food injustice and supports and honors everyone's right to healthy food at all times, and challenges the stigma and shame around food insecurity. URL: https://fooddignitymovement.org/
- **The Food Trust:** works with neighborhoods, institutions, retailers, farmers, and policymakers across the country to ensure delicious, nutritious food for all. Three core programming elements includes access, affordability, and education: https://thefoodtrust.org/
- **Food for Free:** improves access to healthy food through establishing innovative programming and partnerships to overcome barriers and strengthen the community food system. Believes that access to healthy food is a fundamental right. URL: https://foodforfree.org/
- **Foundation for Healthy Schools:** With a mission to reconnect students to the art and science of nature, growing their own produce that will be utilized in school meals, and learning the keys to healthy, nutritious eating. URL: https://foundationforhealthyschools.org/
- **FreshRx:** aims to address nutritional inequality through food programs that provide both education and access to fresh healthy produce, while also supporting local family owned farms that use organic growing practices. URL: https://www.freshrx.org/
- **KidsGardening:** With a mission to create opportunities for kids to play, learn, and grow through gardening, engaging their natural curiosity and wonder, supporting educators and families with resources to get more kids

learning through the garden. URL: https://kidsgardening.org/

- **Urban Gleaners:** picks up fresh food from donors and distributes it to free food markets, schools, and hunger services. Provides a critical link between businesses or farms that have excess food and the food insecure people who need it. URL: https://urbangleaners.org/

- **Wellness in Schools:** a national nonprofit that teaches children healthy habits to learn, live and thrive. Partners with public schools, chefs and coaches to ensure access to nourishing food and active play. URL: https://www.wellnessintheschools.org/

SCIENTIFIC RESEARCH WEBSITES

- **PubMed:** a free database containing more than 37 million citations for biomedical literature from MEDLINE, life science journals, and online books. From the National Institutes of Health (NIH). URL: https://pubmed.ncbi.nlm.nih.gov/

- **ScienceDirect:** 3.3 million articles are published open access, and are peer-reviewed and made freely available for everyone to read, download and reuse. From Elsevier. URL: https://www.sciencedirect.com/

- **Nature:** the world's leading multidisciplinary science journal. Also insightful and arresting news and interpretation of topical and coming trends affecting science, scientists and the wider public. URL: https://www.nature.com/

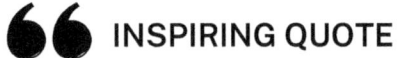 **INSPIRING QUOTE**

"Appreci-eat" your food! Savor the flavor and eat slowly.
It takes your body about 20 minutes to realize it's full."
— Karen Salmansohn

HEALING REVOLUTION DIET: TOP 25 HEALTHY FOODS

This list is simply a starting point. There may be some healthy foods that just do not agree with your gut microbiome – and you shouldn't force them simply because they are healthy. That said, here's a general list of some of the healthiest foods:

- Apples and apple cider vinegar (organic only)
- Avocados and avocado oil
- Beans (kidney, black, lima)
- Beef (grassfed, pastured, regenerative only, including organ meats)
- Berries (strawberries, raspberries, blueberries, blackberries, local or organic)
- Butter (grassfed, pastured, organic only)
- Carrots (local or organic only)
- Chicken (pastured, free range, organic only, including organ meats)
- Citrus (lemons, limes, oranges, local or organic)
- Coffee and teas (organic only)
- Cruciferous vegetables (cauliflower, kale, broccoli, Brussels sprouts, local or organic)
- Eggs (farm-fresh or organic)
- Fermented foods
- Fish (salmon, trout, sardines, wild-caught only)
- Garlic (local or organic only)
- Green beans (local or organic only)
- Mushrooms
- Nuts (walnut, pecan, almond, macadamia, pistachio)
- Olives and olive oil
- Onions (local or organic)
- Potatoes (especially sweet potatoes, non-GMO)
- Seeds (flax, hemp, pumpkin, chia)
- Spinach (local or organic only)
- Watermelons
- Wild meats (bison, elk, venison)

HEALING HINT

Dirt is essential, according to Dr. Josh Axe in his book, *Eat Dirt*. Dirt carries beneficial microbes; we need dirt. "Our bodies crave this dirt, and without dirt, our health is headed in the wrong way."

HEALING REVOLUTION DIET: HEALTHY FOOD CHECKLIST

Here's a list of some of the best foods you can include in your Healing Revolution Diet lifestyle.

Experiment, have fun, and start building your healthy lifestyle!

Best, Healthiest, Nutrient-Dense Proteins

- Pastured, free-ranging (and ideally, local) eggs
- Pastured, grassfed beef (steaks, roasts, ground, organs)
- Wild, free-ranging, pastured elk, one of the leanest natural meats available, with less fat than beef, pork, and chicken (steaks, roasts, ground, organs)
- Wild, free-ranging, pastured bison, also a lean meat (steaks, roasts, ground, organs)
- Wild, free-ranging, pastured venison (steaks, roasts, ground, organs)
- Pastured, free-ranging chicken (whole, cut-up, ground, organs)
- Pastured, free-ranging turkey (whole, cut-up, ground, organs)
- Wild-caught salmon
- Wild-caught trout
- Pastured, grassfed lambs (steaks, roasts, ground, organs)
- Farm-raised pork (steaks, roasts, ground)
- Organic tofu
- Organic tempeh
- Wild-caught sardines
- Wild-caught mackerel
- Organic beans
- Organic lentils

Best, Healthiest, Nutrient-Dense Fats

- Grassfed, pastured butter (ideally from Europe or New Zealand)
- Olive oil (extra-virgin, cold-pressed)
- Avocado oil
- Coconut oil

Best, Healthiest, Nutrient-Dense Fiber Sources

- Mushrooms
- Nuts (pecans, pistachio, macadamia, walnut, hazelnut, Brazil, almond)
- Seeds (chia, hemp, psyllium, flax)
- Avocados (a super food)
- Sweet potatoes (organic)
- Brussels sprouts
- Beans (kidney, black, lima)
- Apples (organic)
- Pears (organic)
- Oranges
- Coffee
- Strawberries (organic)
- Raspberries (organic)
- Blackberries (organic)
- Dried figs, prunes, apricots and dates
- Carrots
- Corn
- Lentils (organic)

Best, Healthiest, Nutrient-Dense Vegetables

- Organic (or farm-fresh) spinach
- Organic (or farm-fresh) kale
- Organic (or farm-fresh) carrots
- Organic (or farm-fresh) broccoli
- Organic (or farm-fresh) asparagus
- Organic (or farm-fresh) sweet potatoes
- Organic (or farm-fresh) Garlic
- Organic (or farm-fresh) Onions
- Organic (or farm-fresh) Brussels sprouts
- Organic (or farm-fresh) green beans
- Organic (or farm-fresh) red or green cabbage
- Organic (or farm-fresh) tomatoes
- Organic (or farm-fresh) bell peppers
- Organic (or farm-fresh) cauliflower

Best, Healthiest, Nutrient-Dense Fruits (in Moderation)

- Organic (or farm-fresh) strawberries
- Avocados
- Watermelons
- Pomegranates
- Organic (or farm-fresh) raspberries
- Organic (or farm-fresh) blackberries
- Organic (or farm-fresh) blueberries
- Organic (or farm-fresh) apples
- Citrus
- Organic (or farm-fresh) red grapes

Best, Healthiest, Nutrient-Dense Omega-3s

- Chia seeds
- Flaxseeds
- Hemp seeds
- Pastured, free-ranging (and ideally, local) eggs
- Wild-caught sardines
- Wild-caught mackerel
- Wild-caught salmon
- Wild-caught herring
- Wild-caught anchovies
- Walnuts

Best, Healthiest, Nutrient-Dense Polyphenol (Including Resveratrol) Foods

- Organic (or farm-fresh) blueberries
- Organic (or farm-fresh) strawberries
- Organic (or farm-fresh) raspberries
- Organic (or farm-fresh) blackberries
- Organic (or farm-fresh) spices (including clove, oregano, sage, rosemary)
- Organic cacao, cocoa powder
- Nuts (especially hazelnuts, pecans, pistachios, and almonds)
- Flaxseed meal
- Coffee and teas
- Olives (both black and green)
- Organic prunes

Best, Healthiest, Mineral-Rich Foods

- Nuts & seeds
- Organic (or farm-fresh) eggs
- Organic (or farm-fresh) organ meats
- Organic (or farm-fresh) cruciferous vegetables
- Mushrooms
- Beans
- Avocados
- Organic Yogurt
- Organic Cheese
- Grassfed beef
- Pastured chicken
- Organic (or farm-fresh) berries
- Wild-caught shellfish

Best, Healthiest Foods With Mitochondrial Boosting Nutrients

- Organic (or farm-fresh) blueberries
- Pomegranate seeds
- Grassfed beef
- Mushrooms
- Broccoli and broccoli sprouts
- Grassfed butter
- Olive Oil
- Wild-caught salmon
- Avocado
- Organic (or farm-fresh) eggs
- Organic (or farm-fresh) spinach
- Flaxseeds

Best, Healthiest, Prebiotic Foods

- Asparagus (organic)
- Avocado
- Bananas
- Beans
- Beets
- Carrots (organic)
- Dandelion greens (organic)
- Garlic
- Honey (organic)

- Jerusalem artichokes (organic)
- Leeks (organic)
- Milk (organic)
- Onions
- Potatoes (organic)
- Root vegetables (organic)
- Tomatoes (organic)

Best, Healthiest, Nutrient-Dense Fermented Foods

- Apple cider vinegar
- Unsweetened (European) Greek yogurt
- Kefir
- Sauerkraut
- Kimchi
- Natto
- Miso

Best, Healthiest, Probiotic Foods

- Apple cider vinegar
- Buttermilk (cultured)
- Cheese (soft)
- Cottage cheese
- Fermented foods (onions, cucumbers, beets)
- Kefir
- Kimchi
- Miso
- Sauerkraut
- Sour pickles
- Turshi
- Yogurt (Greek, plain)

Best, Healthiest, Herbs and Spices

- Basil
- Black peppercorns
- Cardamom
- Cayenne pepper
- Chili powder (capsaicin)
- Cinnamon
- Cloves
- Garlic

- Ginger
- Onion
- Oregano
- Parsley
- Peppermint
- Rosemary
- Sage
- Turmeric

Best, Healthiest, Food Brands

- Ancient Organics
- Amy's Kitchen
- Annie's
- Applegate
- Bai
- Earthbound Farm
- Garlic Gold
- Kerrygold
- Lily's
- Mary's Gone Crackers
- Navitas Organics
- Organic Girl
- Organic Valley
- Pacific Foods
- Primal Kitchen
- Rhythm Superfoods
- Simply Organic
- Simple Truth Organic
- Simple Mills
- Sweetleaf
- Swerve
- Thrive Market
- Vital Farms
- Wholly Guacamole
- Whole Earth
- Wholesome Sweeteners
- Yogi
- Zevia

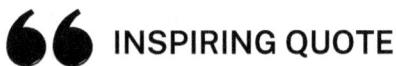 **INSPIRING QUOTE**

"Those who think they have no time for healthy eating will sooner or later have to find time for illness." — Edward Stanley

Healing Revolution Diet: Health, Nutrition, and Diet Glossary

Antioxidants: Critical molecules found in many fruits and vegetables that can help your body neutralize harmful free radicals, which are a normal result of energy production (ATP) from the mitochondria – but become a serious health concern when their levels become too high in your body. When free radicals outnumber antioxidants, it can lead to oxidative stress, which is one of the triggers for multiple health conditions, including death.

ATP: Adenosine triphosphate, the universal energy in all cells, and produced by a process called cellular respiration in the mitochondria, the powerhouse microorganism found in all cells (except red blood cells). ATP is made by converting food into energy. Other functions of ATP include neurotransmission, DNA and RNA synthesis, intracellular signaling, and muscle contraction.

Carbohydrates: One of the historical macronutrients found in foods, along with protein and fat. People should be consuming some carbs, especially for the fiber, but they are not necessary in the enormous quantities being consumed in the Western diet. Carbs can be found in plant-based foods, such as nuts and vegetables. The biggest problem is with ultra-processed foods because food manufacturers have spiked the carb count with starches and huge quantities of added sugar.

Chemicals: In the context of this book, focusing on chemicals as undesirable additives or contaminants used in combination with agriculture and ranching, as well as in the production of many processed foods. Chemicals are not inherently bad, but the overuse and overreliance on chemicals is dangerous. Furthermore, most homes are full of questionable chemicals, from air fresheners to dryer sheets. Our health is being negatively affected by the massive number of chemicals in our lives.

Cholesterol: While it has received a bad reputation and is mostly misunderstood, cholesterol is an important and necessary fat-like substance (lipid) that helps with making cell membranes, hormones, vitamin D, and acids that help you digest foods. In blood tests, it is typically divided into "good" HDL and "bad" LDL cholesterol, but there are now better indicators of cardiovascular disease, such as insulin resistance and diabetes.

Chronic Inflammation: While inflammation is a part of the normal immune system response (such as the bump on your hand after accidentally hitting it), but chronic inflammation is systemic and occurs when the body's immune response becomes excessive and is unable to shut off; it is extremely dangerous and one of the underlying factors in a majority of deaths. Current theories suggest leaky gut – when the protective gut linings weaken and allow toxins into the bloodstream – is a major driver of chronic inflammation. A driver of Leaky Gut is the consumption of ultra-processed and sugary foods.

Conventional Farming: Growing large quantities of crops using heavy machinery and large amounts of chemicals to enhance the soil (mostly nitrogen) and protect against pests (including pesticides and herbicides). The vast majority of corn, soybean, wheat, and fruits and vegetables are grown using conventional methods. Also called factory farming because the goal is to increase yields and profits at all costs, including damaging the soil, hurting the climate, and raising nutrient-weak products.

Conventional Ranching: Typically starts on small farms and ranches until the animals are rounded up into concentrated animal feeding operations (CAFOs) and feedlots. It's in this process in which the process goes awry. Animals are kept in close quarters, for at least 45 days, sometimes indoors, and given an unnatural feed to fatten them up before slaughter. Many are also routinely given antibiotics and growth hormones.

Diet: A way of life, a lifestyle. It should not be a restrictive, painful, time-consuming, calorie-counting, scale-watching experience. Some joke that the word diet is one letter from die. The Healing Revolution Diet is about a lifestyle. All people eating the typical Western or Standard American Diet are leading a way of life that leads to chronic health conditions and early death.

Fat: The most misunderstood and demonized macronutrient found in foods, along with carbohydrates and proteins. Healthy fat is an essential macronutrient that helps the body in several ways, including aiding in the absorption of vitamins and minerals. The largest part of your diet should from healthy fats: grassfed, pastured meats and butter, olives and olive oil, avocados and avocado oil, coconut oil.

Fermented Foods: Our ancestors fermented foods long before refrigeration was invented, and they were probably healthier for it; for them, fermenting was a method of preserving their precious food longer. Today, many people are coming back to fermenting for the health benefits. Fermented foods are produced using bacteria, yeast, or other probiotic-containing organisms to break down sugars, creating unique flavors as well as health-promoting foods.

Fiber: A key ingredient in found many foods that is essential to good health; not a macronutrient, but should be (instead of carbohydrates). Fiber is essential in aiding weight management, blood sugar regulation, and digestion. The beneficial bacteria in the gut microbiome crave fiber, which take it and ferment it to release nutrients for the body and brain. Fiber is found in vegetables and nuts and seeds, as well as fruits and legumes.

Fructose: The worst element of sugar, found in many plants and derived from sugar cane, sugar beets, and corn (high fructose corn syrup). It feeds the bad bacteria in our guts, then gets sent to the liver, where it can lead to fatty liver disease, as well as raising blood triglyceride levels. Because it does not get absorbed, it also negatively impacts the production of leptin, which is a hormone that suppresses appetite, leading people to eat more.

Grassfed: If you are going to eat any meats, it is extremely important to only buy wild or pastured, grassfed, which is the healthiest meats and proteins. Grassfed animals forage their entire lives in pastures, eating their natural diet. Conventionally raised animals are fed unnatural feeds and antibiotics to fatten them for higher profits. But grassfed is a term food marketers have manipulated, so be careful examining labels. The highest certification is the *Certified Grassfed by AGW (A Greener World)*.

Gut Dysbiosis: Occurs when there is an imbalance between beneficial and harmful bacteria in the intestines, which makes the gut more vulnerable to diseases and other health conditions. Dysbiosis often results in the loss of beneficial bacteria and then to a dangerous increase in the harmful bacteria. It can manifest as stomach aches, bloating, heartburn, achy joints. Worse, if left untreated, it leads to a range of chronic illnesses and conditions

Gut Microbiome: The collection of micro-organisms (mostly bacteria, but also viruses, yeasts, and others) that reside chiefly in the intestines, and which play a role in digestion, metabolism, immunity, emotions, and mental health. It is the largest and most important "organ" in our body and it is absolutely essential to have a strong and diverse mix of beneficial bacteria. Sadly, many researchers have shown that our limited food system (because of so many imposter, ultra-processed foods) has caused a number of beneficial bacteria to go extinct. Prebiotics and probiotics both help strengthen the gut microbiome.

Health: The absence of disease/illness while living in a state of physical, mental, emotional, and social homeostasis and well-being. A healthy lifestyle helps lead to a full life, lived with happiness and positivity. The most important factor that affects health is food; invest in healthy, nutrient-rich foods. Poor health, often from a nutrient-poor diet, can lead to both mental and physical conditions.

Healing: A process of acknowledgment, acceptance, forgiveness, and integration of the emotional wounds from painful life experiences/traumas. A healing journey is the exploration and reconciliation of one's entire life. It is necessary for living one's optimal and best life. The journey is not always smooth, and rarely linear, but the insights and understanding and peace received is worth the effort. Often it takes starting a healing journey to realize the importance of a health journey.

Healthspan: Living a long life free from serious and chronic diseases. Longevity is wonderful, but if the average 60+ year-old lives another 20-30 more years filled with one or more chronic conditions that dramatically affect the quality of life, how is that something to aspire to? (Studies show the typical person spends about 20 percent of their lives unhealthy; expect to see that percentage dramatically increase in the next decade.) Healthspan is living a long and healthy life, which is something we should all aspire to.

Imposter Foods: Any food that has been ultra-processed is a fake food. Food scientists at all the major food brands transform the ingredients in the lab, deconstructing to core elements so that they can then be recreated into food-like substances. Imposter foods are high in sugar and have replaced healthy fat with unsafe seed oils (because they are dirt cheap), while "enhancing" the foods with chemical additives, including preservatives, emulsifiers, dyes, and more. To add insult to the actual injury from these dangerous ingredients, the scientists also learned how to strip away the beneficial fiber – because without the fiber, people don't get satiated and buy and eat lots more, which means more profits.

Insulin Resistance: A serious condition in which the body does not respond as it should to insulin, a hormone that's critical for regulating blood sugar levels, resulting in excessive sugar in the blood – which causes the pancreas to produce more insulin. Insulin resistance leads to prediabetes and type 2 diabetes, which then leads to heart disease, strokes, cancers, and dementia. Easily reversible with the Healing Revolution Diet.

Intermittent Fasting (IF): A strategy that cycles between periods of not eating anything and eating normally, with the most common technique ending all foods the first day at 7 pm, then either skipping breakfast entirely, or having a late brunch. Any fast is good, but the ideal window is about 14-16 hours. Fasting rests the digestive system and gives the mitochondria a good shock, which results in fat loss, reduced inflammation, brain growth (neuroplasticity), better health, and increased longevity. Some people do IF weekly, monthly, seasonally; experiment with what works for you – and always remember to hydrate.

Leaky Gut: Also called intestinal permeability, it's when the tight junctions of the gut's protective lining become loosened, typically from one or more ultra-processed foods, infections, toxins, medications, and stress. Once the junctions become loose, harmful bacteria and other toxins can pass through the protective lining and enter the bloodstream. When leaky gut occurs, the immune system goes on overdrive to clear the harmful stuff, which can lead to chronic inflammation and a host of chronic illnesses.

Longevity: Living longer than others. The word comes from the Latin word *longaevitās,* including the roots *longus* (long) and *aevum* (age), which combine into a concept that means as living a long life… living a greater duration of life. Forget the Blue Zones; there are hundreds of places all over the world where people are living longer lives. Longevity is a wonderful concept, except that the definition says nothing about the quality of living, just long living. Healthspan is perhaps a better term, meaning living a long and healthy life, free of most chronic illnesses.

Macronutrients: The traditional way to classify the set of nutrients the body needs to function optimally. The three main "macros" include carbohydrates, protein, and fat. Today, experts still support the key roles fat and protein play in nutrition, but the overabundance of carbohydrates in the typical Western diet has caused a movement to downgrade most carbs, which is why this book focuses on the key reason people need at least some carbs: the fiber.

Metabolic Health: Achieving positive levels of certain metabolic markers that deal with metabolic functioning without medication and thus at low risk of cardiometabolic diseases. The five markers are: waist circumference, glucose (or blood sugar) level, blood pressure, triglycerides, and high-density lipoprotein (HDL) cholesterol.

Metabolic Syndrome: When a cluster of three or more health conditions occurs together, often resulting in obesity and increasing the risk of heart disease, stroke, and type 2 diabetes. A diet high in refined carbohydrates, sugars, and ultra-processed foods – while low on fiber, healthy fats, and protein – can lead to less-than-optimal metabolic health.

Metabolism: Involves all the chemical reactions in your cells that convert food or stored energy into fuel. When people eat, the food is broken down into compounds like amino acids (from protein), fatty acids (from fats), and simple sugars (from carbs), which are absorbed into the bloodstream and to various parts of the body.

Mitochondria: The extremely small micro-organisms that are energy sources within the cells of the entire body (except for in red blood cells), with some cells having thousands of mitochondria. Using a metabolic process, they convert food and air into energy – called ATP. They also help heal, detoxify, and strengthen our immunity.

Non-GMO Project: A non-profit organization that certifies food and products in North America that contain no genetically-modified ingredients, but do not confuse non-GMO with organic. All organic products contain no GMO ingredients, as part of the definition of organic, but organic also protects against the use of dangerous chemicals (pesticides, herbicides, etc.) used in conventional farming. Non-GMO simply means the product contains no genetically-modified (now being listed as bio-engineered) ingredients.

Nutrition: The process by which humans use food to support life. The science of nutrition has changed dramatically in the last several decades, smashing old myths and misunderstandings, such as that meat and animal fats are bad or that eating fat causes fat in the body or that cholesterol in food affects blood cholesterol or even that cholesterol is a good marker for cardiovascular issues. Better nutrition is related to improved health, stronger immune systems, lower risk of chronic diseases (such as diabetes, cancer, and cardiovascular disease), and boosting healthspan.

Obesity: A medical condition that is exploding around the world, especially in children, in which a person has accumulated too much fat in the body. It is a driver of multiple chronic conditions, including heart disease, diabetes, high blood pressure, high cholesterol, liver disease, sleep apnea, and certain cancers. While it is often caused by a combination of extremely poor diet (the typical Western consumption of sugary and ultra-processed imposter foods) and environmental factors (see *obesogens*), *it can be reversed through lifestyle choices; one does not need to take drastic medical measures or pharmaceuticals to achieve a healthier weight.*

Obesogens: These are endocrine-disrupting, hormone-influencing, metabolism-distressing chemicals that influence or promote obesity in humans, and which can be found in everyday household items like food containers, toys, cookware, personal care products, cleaning agents, and medical supplies. There are thousands of these chemicals, with the most common including phthalates, atrazine, organotins, perfluorooctanoic acid (PFOA), and Bisphenol-A (BPA).

Omega-3 Fatty Acids: Healthy fats the body needs for functioning that can be obtained from foods (such as fish, olive oil, wild and grassfed animals) or supplements… or both. Most people eating the Western diet are not getting enough of these essential fats that have been shown to support both heart and brain health. Omega-3s also help reduce inflammation and provide protection for multiple chronic health conditions (Metabolic Syndrome).

Omega-6 Fatty Acids: A key fat the body needs, but one that causes inflammation in the quantities most eating the Western diet consume. Other research suggests it also impacts weight gain. These fats are especially high in "vegetable" seed oils (such as canola, corn, soybean), which are the base of most ultra-processed and fast foods. It is extremely important to have a balance in Omega-3 and Omega-6 fats, but today people eating the Western diet consume as much as 25 times more Omega-6 fats.

Organic: Foods that are produced by methods complying with certain standards for the soil, water, and animal welfare. Organically-produced products cannot use any synthetic chemicals (such as pesticides and herbicides), growth hormones, or antibiotics. No part of the food can be genetically-modified (not being called bio-engineered). The U.S. Department of Agriculture (USDA) supervises the organic certification program for any product using the term. Organic does not mean natural, nor does it mean free of toxic sugars or seed oils.

Pasture-raised: When animals are raised outdoors 24/7 and allowed to forage/feed on their natural diets, such as cows on grass and chickens on grass and grubs. Free-range animals, by definition, only have some access to the outdoors. Pastured-raised animals have a better quality of life overall, and it shows in the nutrition density and flavor of the resulting meat. Conventionally-raised animals are fed grain and grain byproducts, often spiked with antibiotics, because it's a cheap food source (because of government grain and corn subsidies) that fattens/sickens cattle, resulting in higher profits.

Polyphenols: Prebiotic compounds found in plants that exert many health and anti-inflammatory benefits and are especially important to the gut microbiome as well as acting as antioxidants in protecting the mitochondria from free radicals produced in energy production (ATP). They are found in fruits, vegetables, cereals, olives, legumes, cocoa, tea, coffee, and wine. More than 8,000 types of polyphenols have been identified, with flavonoids accounting for around 60 percent of all polyphenols. Berries, cocoa, dark chocolate, nuts, flaxseeds, olives, apples, clove, tempeh, coffee, and tea are some of the best polyphenol foods.

Postbiotics: Bioactive compounds, metabolites, the bacteria produce through fermenting the fiber people consume. The idea of supplementing with postbiotics is simply too new and has not nearly been studied enough to make any firm conclusions. In the meantime, you can increase the amount of useful postbiotics in your gut by increasing your intake of fermented foods.

Processed Foods: Any food that has been manipulated in some way; for example, peeling an apple makes it a processed food. Most food is processed in some way before we consume, unless we are eating a completely raw whole foods diet. Cooking is processing. The concern is not processing, but the ultra-processing food manufacturers started doing in the 1980s to this day of manipulating all the ingredients and then recreating them into something that looks like food we know – which is why it is called *imposter foods*.

Protein: An essential macronutrient made from different combinations of 20 amino acids and which help in the formation, management, and recovery of muscles; it is the most filling of the macronutrients. Studies suggest that a high-protein diet has major benefits for weight loss and metabolic health. Furthermore, most people are not eating enough healthy proteins, especially women in menopause. Most people (adults) should get about 25 to 35 percent of daily foods in the form of protein.

Regenerative Farming/Ranching: Truly the hope for the future of farming because this philosophy/strategy focuses on being in harmony with nature instead of fighting it by adding toxic chemicals to the plants or soil. Regenerative is about enhancing and supporting soil health and the soil's unique microbiome, not only making the soil richer and better for growing but also infusing the crops with minerals and vitamins people can absorb when eating. It protects the soil and helps prevent soil erosion and water runoff/pollution. It is the complete opposite of conventional farming and ranching.

Standard American Diet (SAD): The typical diet that most of the Western world consumes disrupts the body's metabolic equilibrium – and it is the foundational cause of unnecessary and premature deaths, the so-called chronic conditions of diabetes, dementia, cardiovascular disease, strokes, liver and kidney diseases, and many cancers. The SAD is comprised of foods produced with excess bad fats (seed oils), extremely high levels of sugar, and multiple chemical additives – while reducing the beneficial fiber. Most of the SAD foods are also made from conventionally raised produce and meats, which are filled with additional chemicals and dangers.

Sugar: An addictive drug that has toxic effects on the body, brain, gut. The sugar industry's own research more than 60 years ago illuminated the health hazards, but with money and influence, not only have they squelched most of the truth about its danger, they also supported any research that proposed that fat was bad and sugar was safe. In the last 20 years, not only have more health experts stepped up but technology has also advanced. We know now that sugar is a toxin that disrupts the gut microbiome and mitochondria functioning – and that can lead to gut dysbiosis and leaky gut, which then leads to all the chronic and deadly illnesses plaguing humanity.

Ultra-processed Foods: Any foods that have been manipulated using industrial formulations that have high concentrations of sugar and seed oils along with a variety of chemical additives (preservatives, emulsifiers, stabilizers, thickeners, trans fats, colorings, etc.) and ingredients not found in nature (such as high fructose corn syrup). These foods are toxic and are contributing to the rapid decline in health, resulting in a slow death. One rule of thumb people use is to not buy any product with unknown ingredients and that has more than five simple ingredients.

Vegetable (Seed) Oils: Extremely cheap, exceptionally dangerous and inflammatory oils that are high in Omega-6 fats and which are produced through an industrial process that involves high heat, solvents, and bleaches. These oils were originally a by-product that was used for industrial machinery. Food companies put these oils (and especially soybean oil) in all ultra-processed and fast foods because they are extremely cheap due to large government farming subsidies. Named seed oils because the oil is extracted from the seeds of corn, soybean, cotton, sunflower, safflower, peanut, rape seed (canola), and palm.

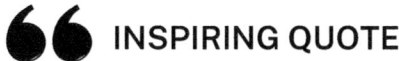 **INSPIRING QUOTE**

"Don't dig your own grave with a knife and spoon."
— English Proverb

HEALING REVOLUTION DIET: FINAL REMINDERS

Here is my parting advice, a handy checklist of what to embrace and what to avoid.

EMBRACE

- Eating more real foods, especially healthy fats and proteins
- Cooking from scratch more often
- Reading food labels carefully
- Choosing healthier ingredients
- Buying locally, then organically, as much as possible
- Consuming more sources of quality fiber
- Eating mindfully
- Feeding and supporting a healthy gut microbiome
- Growing some of your own foods
- Developing quality friends, family, community
- Enjoying more time in nature
- Exercising and movement throughout the day
- Enhancing sleep quality
- Practicing self-care techniques
- Engaging in meaningful work (volunteer or paid)
- Healing from past trauma

AVOID

- All refined sugar (and most processed sugar substitutes)
- Ultra-processed, packaged, takeout, and fast foods
- "Vegetable" seed oils
- Conventionally raised meats, vegetables, and fruits
- Simple carbohydrates
- Most consumption of alcohol and other drugs
- Diets (conventional, fad, etc.)
- Counting calories
- Weighing food
- Stress (especially prolonged periods of stress)
- Most media
- Drama

ABOUT EMPOWERINGSITES.COM

Since 2007, EmpoweringSites.com has been a leader in publishing content that is designed to help people live better lives, starting first with wellness topics before expanding into healing.

The Empowering Sites Network is a content compendium with a mission to help you improve your life... all with free tools, expert advice, and links to the best resources.

EmpoweringSites.com is the corporate parent of several key websites, including:

- HealingRevolutionDiet.com
- HealingSeed.World
- HealMeWhole.com
- TriumphOverTraumaBook.com
- EmpoweringAdvice.com
- MyCollegeSuccessStory.com

EmpoweringSites.com is also the publisher of two books focused on healing:

- *Triumph Over Trauma*
- *Heal!*
- *The Healing Revolution Diet*

We are a small publishing company on a BIG mission of helping the world heal, live their best lives, and foster love and understanding.

Please join us on this mission by healing yourself and then sharing that healing with all the people you know.

To learn more, visit us at EmpoweringSites.com.

YOU CAN HELP EMPOWER OTHERS
TO HEALTH AND HEALING!

If you enjoyed this book and believe others in your community, company, or organization should read it, please consider ordering copies with this special discount!

Retail Price: $17.45

QUANTITY DISCOUNTS

5-20 Books $15.50
21-50 Books $15.00
51-99 Books $14.50
100+ Books $14.00

ORDER YOUR BULK COPIES TODAY!

EmpoweringSites.com
P.O. Box 982
Loon Lake, WA 99148

EmpoweringSites.com

LOOKING FOR OTHER WAYS TO BRING THE HEALING REVOLUTION DIET TO YOUR COMMUNITY?

Contact us today to discuss bringing Dr. Randall's educational and empowering message directly to your community members via a keynote presentation.

ACKNOWLEDGEMENTS

First and foremost, I have a big debt of gratitude for my storytellers; ordinary people who found healing and wanted to share that healing to help others, including **David, Jake, Kali, Chris, Susan, Mandy, Shilpa,** and **Emily.**

Second, I have to thank the nutrition experts who offered advice and tips, **Dr. Linnette Johnson, Tammie Mattos, Jayne Baker, Rebecca Arsena, Janlia Riley, Mandy Rodrigues, Patricia Greenberg, Janelle Cwik, Marica Gaspic Piskovic,** and **Janet Frank, Ph.D.**

Third, I have a special place in my heart for the wonderful people who offered early reviews of the book to help with the marketing of this important project, including: **Lori Shemek, PhD, CNC** and **Dr. Lindy Louise.**

Finally, I have to thank my wonderfully small team who have supported my healing work. First and foremost, the amazing, empathic, and lovely **Jenny Hansen,** a force in the veteran mental health and healing field. Second, the talented book designer, expert sounding board, and just wonderful human, **Michelle Fairbanks.**

WHOLESITIC HEALING BOOK SERIES

The first book in the series.

This book has all the information you need to begin your journey of discovery into whether one or more of these psychedelic medicines may help you. You'll find several chapters covering all the basics of psychedelics – from their fascinating history to how these medicines work to how and what you need to move forward with intentionally using psychedelic medicines – as well as 23 amazingly transformative stories of healing. What are you waiting for?

Transform YOUR life!

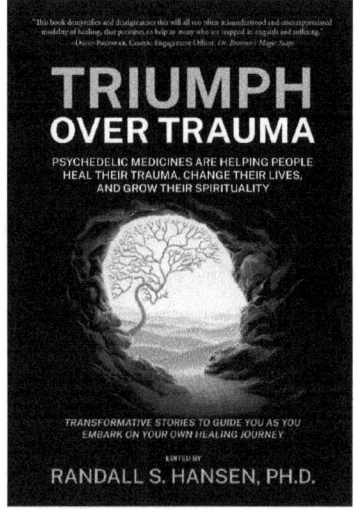

TRIUMPH OVER TRAUMA:
979-8-9872520-0-0

The second book in the series.

This book deconstructs trauma, introduces The Healing Wheel, provides detailed information about the six major modalities of holistic healing, provides key information about finding true healers, reveals healing journey stories, healing fact sheets, and additional wholeistic healing resources. This book is about empowering you to heal yourself, to find yourself, and to live your best life.

It's time to HEAL!

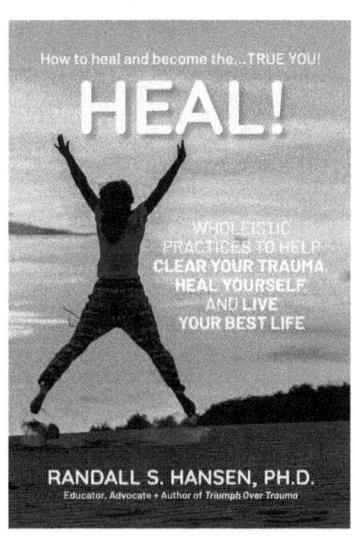

HEAL!
979-8-9872520-2-4

NOTE TO THE READER

Thanks so much for taking the time to join me on this health journey. I hope the words in this book will inspire you to seek true health and healing – for yourself, a loved one, the world.

If the information here speaks to you – and you feel a need to share it – please consider posting a review on Amazon, Barnes & Noble, Goodreads… wherever books are reviewed. And if you do post a review, please share it on social media and tag me (see below).

The more reviews, the more people can find true healing.

Finally, as I hope came across throughout the book, I wish you a beautiful and successful health and healing journey!

DR. RANDALL HANSEN'S CONTACT INFORMATION
WEBSITE: Randallshansen.com
LINKEDIN: Linkedin.com/in/randallshansen
FACEBOOK: Facebook.com/randallshansen/
INSTAGRAM: Instagram.com/empoweringpines/
X (TWITTER): Twitter.com/rshansen/

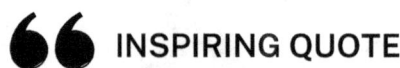

INSPIRING QUOTE

"The food you eat can be the safest and most powerful form of medicine or the slowest form of poison." — Ann Wigmore

EARLY REVIEWS OF
THE HEALING REVOLUTION DIET

The HEALing Revolution Diet book is one of the top resources to help protect and optimize your health. Dr. Randall Hansen provides a customized roadmap to success for you.

Every single aspect of health is science-based and addressed in this groundbreaking book to powerfully change your life.

I highly recommend Dr. Randall's book for anyone looking for serious healthy change.

–**LORI SHEMEK**, PhD, CNC
Award-Winning, Bestselling Author: *How to Fight FATflammation*

"*The Healing Revolution Diet* is a blueprint for anyone looking to create or restore health. This easy read outlines the problems with the modern food environment, how to fix your health by eating real whole foods, and ultimately reduce your dependence on the sickcare system.

Dr. Hansen goes beyond just nutrition and discusses how sleep, self-care, and even the products we use at home contribute to our healing process. This book is part of an ever-growing, larger movement in the mission to take back our health and say goodbye to Big Food and Big Pharma."

–**DR. LINDY LOUISE**, Health consultant
helping people create health by eating real, whole food
YOUTUBE CHANNEL: https://www.youtube.com/@dr.lindylouise

ABOUT THE AUTHOR

DR. RANDALL HANSEN wants you and everyone in the world to find healing and optimal health, living a long and happy life. He shares this passion and Divine mission by educating and empowering people to be proactive about their food choices, find a healthy lifestyle, and heal from past trauma. This book is the third in the Wholeistic Healing Trilogy. He is the author of both the groundbreaking *Triumph Over Trauma: Psychedelic Medicines Are Helping People Heal Their Trauma, Change Their Lives, and Grow Their Spirituality* and the well-received *HEAL! Wholeistic Practices to Help Clear Your Trauma, Heal Yourself, and Live Your Best Life*. Dr. Hansen's focus and advocacy center around true healing ... healing that results in being able to live an authentic life filled with peace, joy, and love. When not writing or educating, you'll find Dr. Randall basking in nature.

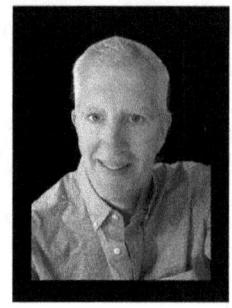

randallshansen.com

www.ingramcontent.com/pod-product-compliance
Lightning Source LLC
Chambersburg PA
CBHW060453030426
42337CB00015B/1569